WHAT TO
DO WHEN
THE DOCTOR
SAYS IT'S

Diabetes

WHAT TO DO WHEN THE DOCTOR SAYS IT'S

Diabetes

The Most Important Things
You Need to Know About Blood Sugar, Diet,
and Exercise for Type 1 and Type 2 Diabetes

WINNIE YU,
MELVIN R. STJERNHOLM, M.D., F.A.C.E.,
and ALEXIS MUNIER

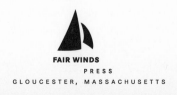

FAIR WINDS
PRESS
GLOUCESTER, MASSACHUSETTS

Text © 2004 Fair Winds Press

First published in the USA in 2004 by
Fair Winds Press
33 Commercial Street
Gloucester, MA 01930

08 07 06 05 04   1 2 3 4 5

ISBN 1-59233-060-6

Library of Congress Cataloging-in-Publication Data available

Cover design: Laura Shaw Design
Book design: *tabula rasa* graphic desugn

Printed and bound in Canada

The information in this book is for educational purposes only.
It is not intended to replace the advice of a physician or medical
practitioner. Please see your health care provider before beginning
any new health program.

I would like to dedicate this book to my loving wife,
Carolyn, who supports me in so many ways.
—Melvin Stjernholm

To mom and dad, whose constant love and support
are always with me in whatever I do.
—Winnie Yu

CONTENTS

INTRODUCTION

As an endocrinologist for more than twenty-five years, I have been on the forefront of some major scientific and medical developments that have changed the way we treat diabetes. I take great pleasure in caring for my diabetic patients, especially when I see them living for many years with the disease, and staying active and healthy. But unfortunately, I am also on the forefront of a national epidemic of diabetes, a situation that I find deeply disturbing, given what I know of the disease.

I first learned about diabetes as a child, watching my grandmother wrestle with this perplexing condition. My grandmother was on insulin until she died at age sixty-three of complications. She never had her blood glucose under control.

Watching my grandmother struggle with diabetes played a big role in my becoming a physician. In the 1960s, as a medical student, I was taught that diabetes was one disease. Back then, everyone thought that adult onset diabetes was strictly inherited and would skip a generation, while juvenile childhood diabetes was passed on to grandchildren. We soon learned that much of this was untrue.

As a medical student, I participated in research that ultimately lead to a better understanding of what causes Type 1 diabetes. Inside medical laboratories, we stimulated the pancreas with glucose, using various chemicals to enhance or inhibit the beta cells in the pancreas to make more or less insulin. We measured insulin using complex double antibody assays with radioactive iodine. Eventually, this type of assay lead to the measurement of other hormones in the bloodstream. Berson and Yarlow eventually won a Nobel Prize for their work in developing insulin antibody technology. Being able to measure insulin helped researchers discover that Type 1 diabetes was a deficiency of the hormone, and that antibodies that attacked beta cells were the cause of the disease.

Still, in the 1970s, the cause of Type 1 diabetes was hotly debated. Autopsy results from a young Type 1 diabetic showed evidence of viral particles in the pancreas. Since Type 1 diabetes occurs more commonly in the fall, when the incidence of all viral illnesses is higher, some scientists postulated that it was caused by a virus. Now we know this is not the case and that Type 1 diabetes is the result of an auto-immune reaction. The viral illnesses combined with the increasing hormones in adolescence makes the disease more common at these peak times.

Prior to the 1900s, we had no treatment for diabetes. We did not understand the cause of diabetes. All we knew was that children who developed this condition would frequently die within days or weeks. Researchers initially thought the hormone that caused diabetes was in the pituitary gland since removal of the gland lowered blood glucose in animals. Later, scientists found that removing the pancreas in animals caused diabetes. Eventually, an extract from the pancreas was used in the treatment of Type 1 diabetes, which was called juvenile onset diabetes because it usually occurred at the beginning of adolescence.

Banting and Best, along with other researchers, were able to isolate crude extracts of insulin from animal sources and give it as injections. Multiple injections of crystalline insulin became the mainstay of treatments. This was a major breakthrough and was the only way to treat diabetes until the 1950s. Insulin products were modified to last longer by adding zinc or protamine, which allowed for once-a-day injections using glass syringes and large needles sharpened with a wet stone at home and sterilized in the oven. By today's standards, this may seem crude, but in the 1920s and 1950s this treatment was prolonging lives by as many as twenty to thirty years.

Today, the Type 1 diabetic often lives fifty to sixty years from the day of diagnosis. This is a dramatic improvement, but does not include Type 1 diabetics with kidney disease, who live only another twenty-five years with the disease if not treated by dialysis or given a transplant.

Finding a way to avoid kidney disease is just one of many medical mysteries left to solve in diabetes. There are plenty of other unanswered questions. For instance, why do some diabetics get kidney disease and not others, even those with poorly controlled blood glucose? Why do some develop eye disease, while others get neuropathy? Why do some manage to escape complications altogether? We still need more answers and better solutions. Scientists are working to find answers to these very intriguing questions.

Ironically, as our knowledge about diabetes has grown in this past century, so too has the incidence of Type 2 diabetes, especially in recent decades. A recent article in *Time* magazine reports that the numbers of people in the U.S. who have diabetes is expected to double by the year 2025. The disease is expected to triple in Africa, the eastern Mediterranean, the Middle East, and Southeast Asia.

An aging population is one reason behind the surge in diabetes, which is more prevalent among adults over the age of fifty. But there are greater numbers of young adults, even teenagers, being diagnosed with Type 2 diabetes. There is no doubt in my mind that the reason for the increase in the disease lies in our lifestyle. We live in an era when people spend their work hours in front of a computer and their free time lounging in front of the television. We live on unhealthy foods and eat them in ever-larger portions. Then, when we gain weight, we struggle with the challenges of dieting, always looking for an easy answer—a gimmicky diet or pill, or gastric bypass surgery—to help us shed those extra pounds, rather than make the necessary lifestyle changes to keep the weight off. Our children are learning these behaviors and gaining weight as well.

Given my own family history, I have personally decided it is time to lose weight and exercise more to prevent myself from developing this disease. After all, I want to live to see my grandchildren graduate from college and have the pleasure of seeing my great grandchildren. In the last three months, I have lost twenty pounds. I feel much better and am less short of breath climbing stairs. I have also learned to eat less and to avoid potatoes, pizza, pasta, white bread, white rice, and bagels, all culprits behind my weight gain. In addition, I am learning to eat smaller portions of meat. Instead of the usual six to eight ounces, I now eat just four ounces. I eat more chicken and fish and less red meat.

For exercise, I work in my yard and run on the treadmill. I now park far from the entrance of a store or supermarket, which allows me to enjoy a short walk. Instead of taking the elevator at work, I climb the stairs. And I am also taking time to enjoy sports I like, namely tennis, golf, and skiing.

I do this not only for myself, but for my patients. In my practice, half my patients have diabetes, and they're evenly split between Type 1 and Type 2. As a physician, I must set a good example of healthy behavior if I am to preach its virtues. And I do preach about the importance of diet and exercise. Lifestyle changes can have a tremendous impact on diabetes. Losing weight can delay the onset of diabetes in more than 80 percent of the population at risk. Maintaining an ideal body weight and simply walking thirty minutes a day may be enough to prevent the disease altogether. These lifestyle changes can even help people who are well on their way to developing Type 2 diabetes or have already been diagnosed. The Diabetes Prevention Program showed that people who have impaired glucose tolerance were able to delay the onset of diabetes by more than 2.8 years with lifestyle changes. In people already diagnosed with Type 2 diabetes, lifestyle changes can delay the need for insulin shots.

We Americans are blessed to live in a prosperous era, with tremendous scientific knowledge and new technological capabilities. Medical advances have greatly enhanced our ability to avoid infectious diseases, which were once a common cause of death before the twentieth century, when most people didn't live beyond age fifty. Today, we can prevent most infectious diseases with immunizations. We can purify our water supplies and prevent pollution of our water with sanitation technology. We have antibiotics to prevent staph and strep infections.

Despite these advances, many still face the ravages of diabetes. But scientific progress has also improved the treatment and control of diabetes. We know, for instance, that eating well and exercising regularly can prevent the onset of diabetes and minimize complications of the disease. We have new insulins and insulin pumps that have revolutionized the daily care involved in diabetes. We have new cholesterol lowering agents and anti-hypertensive agents that can reverse or delay the progression toward kidney disease and other complications of diabetes.

But none of this matters if you do not educate yourself about diabetes. If you've picked up this book, you've taken a giant step toward becoming better educated about diabetes and taking control of your health. Education after all, is the key to good diabetes control and the prevention of complications. *What to Do When the Doctor Says It's Diabetes* will help you and your loved ones understand this complex condition. Diabetes is a disease that raises many questions. I hope you will find your answers in this book.

—Melvin R. Stjernholm, M.D., F.A.C.E.

CHAPTER ONE

Diabetes: What Is It?

By now, you've probably heard about the alarming increase in diabetes in this country. Americans' penchant for unhealthy foods and the lack of physical activity has made this disease so common that it now afflicts approximately six percent of the population, or seventeen million people—more than the number of people living in the entire state of Florida.

Amazingly enough, as many as six million of those people have no idea they even have diabetes. They have no definitive signs or symptoms, no indications that anything is wrong. Or if they do, they chalk it up to advancing age or a hectic lifestyle. Yet, left uncontrolled, the illness could eventually wreak havoc on their bodies, causing conditions as serious as heart disease, blindness, stroke, or kidney failure.

That's why diabetes is aptly named the silent killer, a disease that develops slowly and often with no apparent symptoms. Often, it's years before you realize that something is wrong. By then, it may be too late. The complications have taken their toll.

The good news is, you are among the other eleven million people who know—or at least suspect—you have the disease. Maybe it was too many nightly trips to the bathroom that tipped you off. Or an unquenchable thirst that sent you to the water cooler every ten minutes. Perhaps you noticed blurred vision, recurring infections that were slow to heal or inexplicable weakness and fatigue. Maybe you found yourself gaining or losing weight for no apparent reason. Or maybe, unfortunately, it was a diagnosis of something more serious that lead to the discovery you have diabetes.

Knowing you have diabetes is crucial to your health because it means you can now do something about it. Although diabetes is a serious disease with life-threatening implications, it can be monitored and controlled. And with some lifestyle adjustments, you can still live a long, healthy, productive life.

The key to managing your condition is learning as much as you can about diabetes and then taking good care of yourself. That means eating well, exercising regularly, taking your prescribed medications, and constantly monitoring your blood glucose and getting it to healthy levels. Let's begin by defining what diabetes is and examining the three different types.

What Is Diabetes?

Simply put, diabetes mellitus is a metabolic disorder, a malfunction of the body's ability to use the energy in food. The disease was recognized as early as around 1550 B.C., when early Egyptians noted a condition that involved the passing of too much urine. The ancient Greeks gave it the name diabetes, which means "siphon" or "pass through." In the late eighteenth century, the Latin term mellitus was added to describe the sugary quality of the urine. In fact, an early method of diagnosing diabetes was by pouring urine near an anthill. If the ants flocked to it, it was evidence that the urine contained sugar.

The problems involved in diabetes begin in the way your body derives energy from food. Whenever you eat, food travels to your stomach, where it is broken down into glucose during the digestion process. Glucose, which is the body's primary source of energy and comes mostly from carbohydrates, enters the bloodstream, where it is then referred to as blood glucose or blood sugar. In healthy people, the pancreas responds by releasing the hormone insulin into the bloodstream. Insulin is made by beta cells located in the Islets of Langerhans in the pancreas, which sound like a chain of exotic islands but are in fact the production centers of insulin.

Once the insulin courses through the bloodstream, it behaves like a key, unlocking cells and letting the sugar enter, thereby removing the sugar from your blood. Inside the cells, the sugar is converted into energy that your body uses for everything from running a marathon to folding laundry. If the body doesn't need to use glucose immediately, it can send the excess to the liver or the muscles, where it is stored as glycogen to be used later.

In people who have diabetes, the body no longer responds to the insulin it produces, a condition known as insulin resistance, or it fails to make enough insulin. Either way, the body cannot convert the glucose into energy, and excess sugar lingers in the blood. The excess glucose is eventually eliminated through the urine. But getting rid of the extra sugar wears on the kidneys, which now require more water to flush out the sugar. The result is frequent urination and excessive thirst.

Over time, the repeated buildup of blood glucose starts to take its toll throughout the body. In addition to the wear and tear on your kidneys, other parts of the body can be affected. Here is just a sampling of what excess glucose can damage:

- *Nerves.* Too much sugar interferes with the ability of your nerves to transmit impulses, causing a condition called neuropathy. Nerve damage can result in weak muscles, burning sensations, numbness, tingling, and decreased sensitivity.
- *Blood vessels.* High glucose levels can inflict damage on blood vessels, putting diabetics at greater risk for heart disease, heart attack, and stroke.

- *Immune system.* Too much sugar in the blood blocks your body's natural healing process, making you vulnerable to infections. Common sites for infection include the skin, mouth, lungs, bladder, feet, and genital area.
- *Eyes.* Excess blood glucose can cause the fluid in the lenses of your eyes to dry out, making it hard for you to focus. Over time, it can damage the retinas and cause diabetic retinopathy, a condition that develops over a period of fifteen to twenty years in approximately eighty percent of all diabetics. Left untreated, it can cause blindness.
- *The skin.* The body's extreme demand for fluids typically causes the skin to dry out, leaving it vulnerable to infections.

The Three Kinds of Diabetes

Diabetes is not one single disease, but rather comprised of three different variations. Although all three are characterized by a malfunction in the body's ability to produce energy from glucose, each one occurs for different reasons.

Type 1 Diabetes

Type 1 diabetes, once known as juvenile diabetes, is an autoimmune disorder, in which the body attacks its own healthy cells, in this case beta cells. Once the beta cells are destroyed, the patient becomes dependent on self-administered insulin for survival, which is why the disease used to be called insulin-dependent diabetes. That name was discarded because many Type 2 diabetics also require insulin to maintain blood sugar levels.

Approximately five to ten percent of all cases of diabetes in the United States are Type 1, or approximately one million people. About half are diagnosed before the age of twenty, though some patients may develop it after age thirty. Men and women are equally afflicted, but the condition is more common in whites than non-whites. And for reasons that remain a mystery, the disease is more prevalent among certain northern European countries such as Finland and Sweden. Type 1 diabetes will occur in approximately 1 in 500 children in the United States.

Understanding the risks for Type 1 diabetes is difficult since no one knows exactly what causes the immune system to attack the beta cells in the pancreas, but one thing seems clear: there is no single event that determines whether someone develops Type 1 diabetes. Instead, it appears to be a complex mix of autoimmunity, genetics, and the environment.

Autoimmunity

In healthy people, the immune system guards against disease by killing foreign cells through the action of lymphocytes known as T cells. In people with Type 1 diabetes and other autoimmune disorders, the actions of the immune system have gone amok. Rather than attack foreign invaders, the lymphocytes go after the body's own healthy cells. They do it with the guidance of substances known as autoantibodies.

Researchers have found that people who have Type 1 diabetes are more likely to have autoantibodies that can recognize islet cells in the pancreas, insulin, and glutamic acid decarboxylase or GAD, a protein made in the pancreas by the beta cells. These antibodies spearhead the destruction of the insulin-producing beta cells by identifying them for a T cell attack.

Genetics

The genetics of Type 1 diabetes are very complicated, depending on which parent has the disease and when the parent was diagnosed. A child whose father has Type 1 diabetes has a one in seventeen chance of developing the disease. If your mother has Type 1 diabetes and you were born before she was twenty-five years old, your odds are one in twenty-five. If you were born after she was twenty-five, your risk is one in one hundred.

Whether you develop Type 1 diabetes also depends on when your parents were diagnosed. If your parent was diagnosed before the age of eleven, your risk is doubled. And if both parents have Type 1 diabetes, you have a one in ten to one in four chance of getting Type 1 diabetes.

Although scientists have not uncovered a single gene that predicts the onset of Type 1 diabetes, they have found diabetes susceptibility genes. These genes, which are responsible for the functioning of human leukocyte antigens or HLAs, provide the coding information that identifies a person's cells as that of her own. Researchers believe that in people with Type 1 diabetes, the HLAs have misidentified the beta cells in the pancreas as foreign cells or invaders. The immune system then launches an attack that destroys the insulin-producing beta cells. These susceptibility genes are linked to chromosome number 6, which is responsible for autoimmunity.

Several kinds of HLA genes exist, but 95 percent of people with Type 1 diabetes carry the HLA-DR3 form, the HLA-DR4 or both. But genetics are only part of the equation. Many people who have these gene variants do not have Type 1 diabetes. That's why scientists suspect the environment plays a role in triggering the disease, too.

The Environment

When an identical twin gets Type 1 diabetes, his twin sibling has at most a 50 percent chance of developing the disease. The fact that one twin has such a high chance of escaping Type 1 diabetes suggests that other factors are at work in determining who gets Type 1 diabetes.

Exposure to certain viruses such as the Coxsackie virus for instance, is one possibility. The onset of Type 1 diabetes often follows a virus outbreak. The virus theory is bolstered by the fact that Type 1 diabetes typically emerges more frequently in the winter, when more viruses are circulating.

Another possible cause now under scrutiny is early exposure to cow's milk. Conflicting results as to whether a protein in cow's milk can cause Type 1 diabetes has prompted a multinational study launched in 2002 that will examine the role of proteins in cow's milk in genetically at-risk infants. The infants will be monitored for Type 1 diabetes for up to ten years.

In addition, some scientists speculate that oxygen-free radicals may contribute to the onset of Type 1 diabetes. These highly reactive molecules have been implicated in several other diseases, including cancer and atherosclerosis. Certain drugs and chemicals, such as pentamidine, which is used to treat pneumonia and pyriminil, a rat poison, are also known to trigger Type 1 diabetes.

Type 2 Diabetes

In most people who have Type 2 diabetes, the pancreas continues to manufacture insulin, but the body's cells no longer respond to it, a condition known as insulin resistance. In other patients, the pancreas has stopped making insulin or fails to produce enough to get the glucose out of the blood. Either way, the glucose can't get into the body cells for conversion into energy and is left to accumulate in the bloodstream.

Like Type 1 diabetes, Type 2 does have a genetic connection. If you had a parent with Type 2 diabetes, your odds for developing the disease are one in seven if the parent was diagnosed before age fifty. The odds go up to one in thirteen, if your parent was diagnosed after age fifty. If both parents have Type 2 diabetes, you have a 50 percent chance of getting it, too. The condition is also more common in African Americans, Native Americans, Asian Americans, Hispanic Americans, and Pacific Islanders.

The genetic link is actually stronger in Type 2 diabetes than it is in Type 1 diabetes. An identical twin whose sibling develops Type 2 diabetes has a 75 percent chance of getting the disease, compared to a 50 percent chance in Type 1 diabetes. But lifestyle factors also play a much bigger role in the development of Type 2 diabetes and may actually override the genetic influences. Those include:

Being Overweight

As many as 90 percent of all diabetics are overweight. Excess amounts of fatty tissue makes your body cells less sensitive to the effects of insulin, especially if the weight is concentrated in the stomach rather than the hips and thighs. And if you're obese—defined as weighing 20 percent more than you should—your risk is 7.5 times greater than someone who is at a normal weight.

Lack of Exercise

Without regular exercise, you are automatically at risk for diabetes. Physical activity works on several levels to keep the condition at bay. It controls your weight, promotes the use of blood sugar for energy, makes muscle cells more sensitive to insulin, and improves blood circulation. Exercise also helps build muscle mass, which absorbs sugar from the blood.

High Saturated Fat, High Sugar Diet

Americans have become famous for eating unhealthy diets. Foods that promote weight gain and obesity make you more vulnerable to Type 2 diabetes.

Other Risk Factors

Beside your lifestyle, other factors can raise your chances of developing Type 2 diabetes. For instance, you're also at greater risk if you had gestational diabetes while you were pregnant or delivered a baby who weighed more than nine pounds.

Simply getting older can elevate your chances of developing Type 2 diabetes, too. As we age, we tend to become less active, lose muscle, and gain weight. Nearly one in five Americans aged sixty-five or older has diabetes. But in recent years, the disease has become more common among younger adults as the prevalence of weight gain and inactivity has increased.

Some health conditions can put you at risk for developing Type 2 diabetes as well. People who have high blood pressure—defined as greater than 140/90 mmHg in adults—are more likely to get Type 2 diabetes. Low levels of HDL cholesterol, the good cholesterol, below 35 mg/dL, and high trigylceride levels of 250 mg/dL or more can also put you at greater risk. Women who have polycystic ovarian syndrome have a higher likelihood of developing Type 2 diabetes, too, because the condition is related to insulin resistance.

Gestational Diabetes

As the name suggests, gestational diabetes occurs during pregnancy. About two percent of all pregnant women, or 135,000 patients, develop this condition each year.

In women who develop gestational diabetes, their bodies cannot make enough insulin or use the insulin they need, which causes blood sugar levels to rise. Placental lactogen, a hormone made by the placenta, combined with a genetic predisposition for diabetes, is believed to play a role in causing the insulin resistance that occurs in gestational diabetes.

Some women are at greater risk for gestational diabetes. Women who are older than twenty-five, overweight before conception, and who have a family history of diabetes are more likely to develop the disease. Non-white women appear to be at greater risk than white women. And women who have given birth to large babies or who were themselves nine pounds or larger at birth seem to be at greater risk.

The good news is that gestational diabetes is usually a temporary condition and almost always disappears after delivery. But the woman is at higher risk for developing Type 2 diabetes later in life.

Like Type 2 diabetes, gestational diabetes may occur with few or no symptoms. For instance, the constant need to urinate is a common problem of pregnancy and does not necessarily signal that anything else is wrong. Fatigue, another symptom in pregnancy, may be an indication of gestational diabetes. That's why doctors routinely perform an oral glucose tolerance test sometime between the twenty-fourth and twenty-eighth weeks of pregnancy, when pregnancy hormones escalate and begin to interfere with the function of insulin.

How Do I Know I Have Diabetes?

When someone has Type 1 diabetes, the symptoms develop quickly and are usually so severe that the patient knows something is wrong. But for people who have Type 2 diabetes, the disease can linger in the body for years with no apparent symptoms. Nightly trips to the bathroom are simply considered a nuisance and ignored, and fatigue may be chalked up to a busy lifestyle. Gestational diabetes is difficult to distinguish from the normal symptoms of pregnancy.

When the symptoms do emerge, they are usually similar and may include:

- *Frequent urination.* People with diabetes may urinate up to twenty times a day, with a full bladder every time. That's because the kidneys are working overtime trying to rid the body of the excess glucose. In the process, the extra sugar soaks up water throughout the body, causing frequent urination.
- *Extreme thirst.* As the excess sugar absorbs water, the body dehydrates, and the patient becomes extremely thirsty. People with Type 1 diabetes may drink gallons of water a day and still feel thirsty.
- *Unexplained weight loss.* Because body cells aren't getting the energy they need from food, the body begins to break down fat and muscle for energy. In some Type 1 diabetics, the weight loss may occur despite an increase in appetite as the body makes a futile effort to correct the energy deficiency.
- *Weight gain.* Your cells are starved for energy, so you eat more to compensate, which in turn causes you to gain weight.

- *Fatigue and weakness.* Without the ability to produce energy in your body cells, diabetics often suffer from chronic fatigue.
- *Flu-like symptoms in Type 1 diabetes.* In Type 1 diabetics, these symptoms may indicate diabetic ketoacidosis, a condition characterized by high levels of ketones in the urine. Ketones are toxic chemicals produced when the energy-starved body begins to break down fat for energy. High levels of ketones can cause the following: fever; nausea; vomiting; deep, rapid breathing; and loss of appetite. Left unchecked, ketoacidosis can become fatal.
- *Blurred vision.* When the high levels of sugar in your blood pull fluid from the lenses of your eyes, the result is often an inability to focus.
- *Slow-healing cuts and infections.* The sugar-rich blood makes it hard for your white blood cells to fight off infections. As a result, cuts and scrapes, especially on your skin and gums, take longer to heal.
- *Numbness and tingling.* Once the excess blood glucose has started to damage your nerves, you may experience numbness or tingling in your hands or feet. Sometimes, you may feel a burning sensation in your extremities.
- *Yeast infections.* This is a common problem for many diabetic women. Candida, the most common type of microscopic fungus behind most yeast infections in humans, thrives in a high-sugar environment.

Diagnosing Diabetes

Doctors rely on several different tests to confirm whether you have diabetes. They include:

- *Fasting plasma glucose test.* After an overnight fast, a sample of blood is drawn for laboratory analysis. Normal levels are less than 100 milligrams per deciliter (mg/dl). If your fasting plasma glucose levels are more than 126 mg/dl on two or more tests on different days, you are said to have diabetes.

- *Random plasma glucose test.* Samples of blood drawn shortly after eating or drinking may also be used to test for diabetes. Blood glucose levels above 200 mg/dl suggest diabetes, but a fasting plasma glucose or oral glucose test must be done to confirm the results.
- *Oral glucose tolerance test.* Following an overnight fast of at least eight hours but no more than sixteen hours, your blood is drawn for analysis. After that test, you are given 75 grams of glucose in a syrupy drink. Blood samples are then drawn up to four times in the next two to three hours. A healthy person will have blood glucose levels below 140 mg/dl at all intervals.
- *Urine test.* While the urine test is not generally used for diagnosis, excess levels of blood glucose do turn up in the urine. A urine test is also helpful in detecting high levels of toxic chemicals called ketones, made when the body is breaking down fat for energy.

The Current Epidemic

These days, diabetes has become a major health crisis in the United States, a trend that directly parallels the stunning increase in the numbers of overweight and obese people. By some estimates, there are 2,700 people diagnosed each day, with approximately a million new cases a year.

Among the most disturbing trends is the increase in the numbers of children and adolescents being diagnosed with Type 2 diabetes. The Centers for Disease Control and Prevention predicts that one out of every three Americans born after 2000 will develop diabetes.

Who are these children? According to the American Diabetes Association, as many as 80 percent of the children with Type 2 diabetes are overweight. Most are older than ten years of age, but the disease has been documented in kids as young as four. The children also tend to have a family history of Type 2 diabetes and are frequently members of an ethnic group, such as Native American, African American, or Hispanic American.

Similarly, as the nation becomes increasingly overweight and obese, diabetes is also becoming more common among younger adults. In 2000, approximately 28 percent of adults with the disease said they were diagnosed when they were younger than forty, which puts them at greater risk for future illnesses, such as heart disease and stroke. One study found that young adults aged 18 to 44 who develop Type 2 diabetes are 14 times more likely to have a heart attack and 30 times more like to have a stroke than their healthy peers.

The ramifications of this epidemic are enormous. Diabetes may be only the fifth leading cause of death in the United States, but it contributes to the development of heart disease, stroke, hypertension, blindness, and kidney disease—all potentially life-threatening conditions.

Economically, diabetes is exacting an enormous toll. The total cost of diabetes in 2002 was about $132 billion, or one out of ten health care dollars spent in the U.S. Of that, $92 billion was spent on direct medical costs, with the rest in indirect costs such as disability, work loss, and premature mortality. Individually, people with diabetes spent an average of $13,243 in 2002, compared with healthy people whose health care expenses totaled $2,560.

A Note on Pre-Diabetes

At least another sixteen million people in the U.S. have a condition called pre-diabetes, also called impaired glucose tolerance. These people have blood sugar levels that are higher than normal, but not high enough to be diagnosed with diabetes. On blood tests, their glucose levels are higher than 100 mg/dl, but less than 126 mg/dl. The range was recently lowered from 110 mg/dl to 100 mg/dl, in the hopes that more people will take action before the condition worsens.

While pre-diabetes is not the same as Type 2 diabetes, it is considered a serious medical problem. People with pre-diabetes are 1.5 times more likely to get cardiovascular disease than their healthy peers and have a higher chance of heart attack and stroke. And without intervention, they will most likely develop Type 2 diabetes in ten years.

Anyone who is over forty-five years of age and overweight should be tested for pre-diabetes. You should also be tested if you have other risk factors, such as a family history of the disease, high cholesterol, high blood pressure, or a history of gestational diabetes.

The good news is, people with prediabetes can prevent or delay the onset of Type 2 diabetes by changing their lifestyle. Exercising thirty minutes a day and losing as little as ten to fifteen pounds can help slow the progress of the disease. In some people, the condition can even be reversed, as blood glucose levels go back to normal.

Is There Any Hope?

Given the grim statistics, it might appear we're doomed to live with diabetes and to accept its inevitable consequences as fate. But that's far from the truth. Experts now know that making small changes in your lifestyle can help prevent the disease even in people who are at high risk for Type 2 diabetes. By exercising, eating right, and being vigilant about your weight, cholesterol levels, and blood pressure, you may be able to stave off diabetes for years, even for good.

And for people who already have diabetes, taking charge of your health can bring blood glucose levels under control and put you on the path to a healthier life. All it takes is a commitment to making some lifestyle changes, like losing weight, eating better, and getting more exercise. You will also need to take your medications, monitor your blood sugar levels, and be extra vigilant about your overall health.

No, it won't be easy. For some, these changes may require tremendous effort. For others, it may mean a serious overhaul of old habits. But in the end, the rewards of a healthy life will be well worth it.

A PERSONAL STORY

Sabrina

For Sabrina, one of the first symptoms of diabetes was the throbbing headaches. Nothing she took relieved them, and Sabrina simply blamed them on her job. "I was putting in long hours, and initially attributed my headaches to work," says Sabrina, forty-one, a human resources planner.

Then there was the overwhelming fatigue, the unquenchable thirst, and the frequent need to urinate. Going to the bathroom as often as ten times a night only made her more tired. At work, colleagues took steps to accommodate her problems. She had a pitcher of water delivered from the cafeteria to her office every forty-five minutes, and the human resources manager put an out of order sign on the bathroom closest to her, so she had quick access any time she had to go.

Sabrina suspected she might have diabetes. After all, she already had three major risk factors before her symptoms even developed: she was overweight, an African American, and had family members—her mom, sister, and nephew—who had diabetes. Sabrina decided to get checked out. She made an appointment with her doctor, but then cancelled it when her work load got too busy again.

Sabrina paid a price for not getting to the doctor sooner. One day, before her scheduled appointment, her breathing became irregular. "I was so tired that I was very labored at the slightest task," she says. "Our plant physician called my office regarding a worker's compensation case and realized something was wrong and started asking me questions about symptoms. He said it sounded like I was having difficulty breathing and asked if I'd been drinking more liquids or going to the bathroom more frequently than usual. He told me to come to his office immediately, and I agreed."

Even at that point, Sabrina decided to wait until she completed the report she was working on. But within five minutes, the doctor arrived at her office and insisted she go with him for a checkup. "My gait was unsteady as we walked over there, and he held my arm for support," she says. "I remember seeing the medical office, but not going in. Apparently, I was pretty out of it, and he and the nurses helped me get in the office. They took my sugar reading, and it was about 500. They started an IV, then rushed me to the hospital."

In the hospital, Sabrina was given insulin and put on a diabetic meal plan. She was also told she needed to lose weight. Upon discharge three days later, she was given a prescription for Glucophage. On her own, she attended a diabetes class to learn more about the disease and how to manage it.

When Sabrina got her blood glucose under control, she stopped using the Glucophage and relied just on diet and exercise. And except for a bout of the flu, when rising blood sugars put her back on Glucophage, Sabrina has been able to keep her blood glucose fairly well under control.

These days, good discipline is usually enough for Sabrina to keep her diabetes well controlled. She has lost fifty pounds by watching her fat intake, sticking with lean meats, and limiting her consumption of dairy foods. She writes out a weekly menu that follows diabetic dietary guidelines, and exercises three times a week by walking on a treadmill and doing an exercise tape. "When I exercise regularly and eat properly, I show no signs of diabetes, unless I work through my lunch hour, and my glucose drops too low," she says. "I keep medication around for when it's high, glucose tablets for when it's low. And I keep peppermints in my purse, glove compartment, and desk drawer for emergencies."

Sabrina says she should have gotten tested sooner than she did, especially with all the symptoms she had. "People know their bodies, but they have to take action on what their bodies are saying," Sabrina says. "Any time you're drinking as much water and going to the bathroom as much as I was, you'll know. The sooner you know you have diabetes, the sooner you can treat it."

CHAPTER TWO 🐟

Picking a Medical Team

Anyone who has ever played a group sport knows the importance of picking a good team. You want the best player for each position. Then, if every player does his best, the whole team succeeds.

Putting together a medical team to help you treat and manage your diabetes is done in a similar way. You want to select the best health-care professionals to handle every aspect of your health, be it your feet, your teeth, or your mental well-being.

As you already know, diabetes is incredibly complicated and can affect so many aspects of your health, literally from head to toe. It can cause several kinds of infections, difficulties in your eyesight, and problems in your blood vessels and vital organs. That's why one doctor is not enough. No one physician can possibly detect or treat the range of health complications you might encounter, nor would he even attempt it. A team approach to treating your diagnosis of diabetes is a must.

For many people, however, the task of finding so many medical professionals may seem daunting. Until now, you may have relied on just one doctor for all your health-care needs. Sure, you may have gone to the dentist once or twice a year and seen an eye doctor occasionally.

If you're a woman, you also probably have an obstetrician/gynecologist. Maybe you made an occasional visit to a specialist like an allergist or dermatologist.

But having diabetes means you'll need more medical attention than you did before because the disease affects virtually every system in your body. It may also create emotional and psychological issues that you've never experienced, and involve medications and lifestyle changes that can seem overwhelming.

Assembling a good medical team is of critical importance. These are the people who will help you develop a custom plan to manage your condition and keep you as healthy as possible. In this chapter, we'll look at the key players on your medical team, the specialists who might be called to action, and the unique roles they'll play.

Who's in Charge?

The answer is easy: you are. Consider yourself the coach of this evolving medical team. Sure, your primary care doctor may give you the names of some good diabetes doctors. Or you may get referrals from your friends and family. But ultimately, you must decide whom you will enlist.

The key is knowing what you want in a health-care provider. Do you want someone whose office hours match your work hours? Do you want someone with a gentle approach or a less personal one? Would you prefer to work with someone who's been in practice a long time or someone who is relatively new to the field of health care? Only you can answer those questions.

The American Diabetes Association suggests looking for medical professionals who satisfy the three Rs:

- *Recognize.* Do they recognize you as an individual and allow you to give input into your care?
- *Respond.* Do they respond openly to your questions and concerns?

Do they give you the time and attention that you might require?
Are they clear in their conversations?
• *Recommend.* Do they make good recommendations for your care?

Choosing the members of your medical team also involves some personal chemistry. You want to select health-care professionals you respect and trust, whose advice and directions you will follow. After all, if you don't respect your doctor, you will be less likely to follow his directions and take your medications.

You also need people who put you at ease, so that you can freely share any concerns, no matter how personal they may be. Some of the problems associated with diabetes are sexual. Others may be emotional. For some people, these are difficult topics to talk about if they're unaccustomed to sharing details of their lives with acquaintances. But when it comes to managing your diabetes, you need to talk about anything that concerns you and your health.

So make sure to select a medical professional who makes you comfortable. If your gut instinct signals that something isn't right, you should probably keep looking around. Next, we'll look at the people you will need on your team.

The Lead Doctor

To help you manage your blood glucose levels and to oversee your overall health, you will need a physician who acts as your primary treatment provider. This primary care doctor may be an internist, a family practitioner, a general practitioner, or a diabetologist. Diabetologists are medical doctors who have a special interest in treating diabetes.

You may want to consider enlisting an endocrinologist. Endocrinologists are medical doctors who specialize in diseases affecting the endocrine system, which regulate the hormones in your body. Diabetes is an example. Endocrinologists are board certified in internal medicine and then take three years of training in the subspecialty of endocrinology, diabetes, and metabolism. They are trained to manage the complexities of diabetes when the primary care physician cannot control your diabetes adequately or is not able to answer your questions. Most endocrinologists no longer do primary care, but are happy to work closely with your primary care provider.

Ideally, your primary care physician should be well-versed in diabetes care and stay abreast of developments in the disease, including new research, treatments, and information about managing diabetes. This person will help you with the medical management of your condition, offer suggestions for choosing the other members of your medical team, and keep on top of any complications that might develop.

It's always a good idea to conduct an informal interview of a medical professional before you agree to be a patient, especially when it's the lead doctor overseeing your diabetes care. You are in effect, hiring that person to do the all-important job of taking care of you. The process is especially important if you've been diagnosed with diabetes, which may require more frequent medical attention.

Here are some questions you might want answered in your first meeting:

- Does the doctor specialize in diabetes? Where did he or she attend medical school? Is the doctor board certified in internal medicine? Board certification means that beyond medical school, the doctor received at least another three years of training in a specialized field, such as endocrinology, internal medicine, or family practice.
- Does the doctor already have patients with diabetes? If so, what percentage of the patients have diabetes? Are there others who have problems similar to yours? In general, a doctor who already treats patients with diabetes will be better equipped to treat you.

- What kinds of alliances does the doctor have with other health-care professionals who treat diabetes? Are those experts working at the same practice? Is the doctor affiliated with a well-respected hospital? Ideally, your doctor should be able to point you to well-qualified people to help you manage the disease.
- What kind of communications skills does the doctor demonstrate? Does the doctor communicate openly and honestly about your condition? Does he listen to your questions and answer them in a way that you can understand?
- What kind of health insurance does the doctor accept? Diabetes can be costly, and doctor visits may be frequent.
- Is the office conveniently located near your home or office? Is it easy to get appointments?
- Does the doctor seem open to involving you in your health-care decisions?
- How does your doctor feel about your getting a second opinion?
- Finally, did you feel comfortable with the doctor? The complications of diabetes can often be personal, so you want a lead doctor who puts you at ease and with whom you can openly discuss your concerns.

Certified Diabetes Educator (CDE)

Just as the name implies, diabetes educators are people trained to teach you more about your condition. A diabetes educator may be a physician, registered nurse, registered dietitian, pharmacist, exercise physiologist, or social worker.

To become a certified diabetes educator, a health-care professional must be well-versed on physiology, drug treatment, blood glucose testing, complications, mental health issues, and teaching principles. A CDE must also pass a national test, with re-certification exams required every five years. The letters CDE after the name indicates the person is specially trained to work with people who have diabetes.

Diabetes educators are trained to help you learn more about diabetes and guide you on the path to self-care. They can help you determine ways to monitor your blood sugar levels, recognize changing symptoms that require medical attention, and cope with the disease when the stress of it becomes overwhelming.

Dietitian (RD)

One of the most important parts of managing your diabetes is having a well-balanced diet. That's where the registered dietitian comes in. All RDs are trained to understand food and nutrition, but some specialize in diabetes care. Having a registered dietitian on your team will ensure that you devise a well-balanced meal plan that suits your tastes and lifestyle, so that your blood glucose levels do not spin out of control.

In choosing a dietitian, look for the initials RD at the end of his or her name. That means they have met the standards set by the American Dietetic Association and passed a national credentialing exam.

Dietitians will work with you on several fronts to ensure you follow a healthy diet. They can teach you how to count carbohydrates—also called carb counting—as a way to maintain blood sugar levels. They can create an eating plan that will help you lose weight. They can teach you techniques that may adjust your dosage of insulin. In addition, they can help you jazz up a boring diet, adjust your meals to accommodate a new exercise plan, and help you learn to read and understand nutrition labels. Dietitians also can provide recipes, cookbooks, and materials on how to prepare healthy meals.

Eye Doctor

Because diabetes can cause problems in your vision, it's important that an ophthalmologist or optometrist be part of your medical team. Ophthalmologists are medical doctors trained to treat eye problems with surgery or medications. Optometrists, though they can detect eye problems caused by diabetes, cannot do surgery to correct retinopathy, a disease of the retina that is caused by the disease.

A good ophthalmologist will be vigilant in detecting retinopathy, which occurs when blood vessels that fortify the retina, the part of the eye that produces visual images, are damaged. Left untreated, retinopathy can destroy your vision. Ophthalmologists should also be on the lookout for glaucoma, a condition in which the fluid in the eye builds up and causes excessive pressure that can lead to retinal damage. Glaucoma is more common among diabetics than healthy people.

If you are diabetic and over thirty years of age, you should see an eye doctor once a year for a routine exam. Patients who are ten to thirty years old and have had diabetes for at least five years should follow the same schedule. You should also consult an ophthalmologist if:

- You notice changes in your vision, such as blurring, floaters, or spots.
- You experience pain or persistent redness in your eyes.
- Another doctor detects higher pressure in your eyes or retinal abnormalities. High pressure may indicate glaucoma, and retinal changes may be a sign of problems with the retina.

Pharmacist

Before you were diagnosed with diabetes, your relationship with your pharmacist—if you even had one—may have been fleeting. You gave him your prescription, he gave you the medication. With diabetes however, your relationship will become more critical to your well-being.

Pharmacists are trained in the chemistry of drugs and how they affect the body. Finding a regular pharmacist you like is important because that person will have a file of all the medications you take. If you're prescribed a new medication, the pharmacist can alert you to unpleasant side effects and potentially dangerous interactions. You can also turn to your pharmacist for information about the combination of over-the-counter drugs with diabetes medications, whether to take a drug on an empty stomach, and whether you should avoid the sun or certain foods while taking a particular medication.

Foot Doctor

People with diabetes are vulnerable to a variety of foot problems. Poor circulation and damage to the nerves can cause ulcers, deformities, and infections. As many as 15 percent of all people with diabetes will eventually have a foot problem.

That's where the foot doctor or podiatrist comes in. Podiatrists have a Doctor of Podiatric Medicine (DPM) degree and are able to perform surgeries and prescribe medicines to treat your feet. Anything that afflicts your feet, from warts to numbness, comes under the care of a podiatrist. A podiatrist can also show you how to clip your toenails to minimize the risk of infection and point you to shoewear specialists who can help you find well-fitted shoes.

Dentist

Chances are, you already see a dentist once or twice a year for a regular cleaning. Now that you have diabetes, you should visit your dentist every six months. Be sure to tell him you have been diagnosed with diabetes, so he can be on the lookout for any changes in your gums.

Having diabetes makes your mouth vulnerable to infection. Not only is your body less capable of fending off an infection, but the bacteria in your mouth thrive in a high glucose environment. Controlling your blood sugar and having a regular cleaning by a dentist or dental hygienist can keep those bacteria at bay.

In addition to your routine visits, be sure to call your dentist if you see any signs of gum disease, such as bleeding, redness, or swelling. You should also call if you notice a change in your bite, a persistent bad taste in your mouth, or that the gums have pulled away from your teeth.

Other Experts You Might Need:

Dermatologist

Diabetes can wreak havoc on the skin, causing it to dry out or develop fungal and bacterial infections. These conditions require the attention of a dermatologist, a doctor trained in treating skin problems.

Exercise Physiologist

If you'd like to plan a safe, effective exercise program, consider hiring an exercise physiologist. These professionals are scientifically trained to help you devise a program that will help you maintain your blood sugar levels. They may be especially helpful if it's been years since you exercised. Before starting any activity, always check with your doctor.

Mental-Health Professional

Diabetes is a chronic condition, meaning it will never go away. Trying to manage it can be exhausting and frustrating. The result may be chronic stress and feelings of anger, denial, and loss of self-worth. Diabetes can also cause anxiety and depression.

Finding a mental-health professional to help you work out these emotions can help. These professionals may be social workers, psychologists, psychiatrists, or counselors. Besides providing a forum for you to vent, they can also recommend medications, psychotherapy, or both.

It's especially important to treat depression as soon as possible. Depression can interfere with your desire to take care of yourself, which will only make your condition worse.

Kidney Doctor or Nephrologist

The kidney is affected in approximately 35 percent of Type 1 diabetics and 40 percent of Type 2 diabetics. When the kidney is affected by diabetes, it is called diabetic nephropathy. If the kidneys show progressive damage, a kidney specialist or nephrologist should be consulted to make sure the diagnosis is accurate and the treatment is appropriate. Nephrologists are doctors of internal medicine who have also spent three years training in nephrology. They are certified in both internal medicine and nephrology. The endocrinologist is also trained to treat the kidney complications of diabetes, but is not trained to do dialysis or treat end-stage renal disease (ESRD).

Your First Visit

The first time you see your primary care doctor, you will go through a thorough exam that essentially covers your entire health history. The four parts of your visit will involve:

Your Medical History

Usually, this begins with a lengthy questionnaire that asks you to describe your own medical past as well as that of close family members. You may also be asked about lifestyle habits such as smoking, consumption of drugs and alcohol, and allergies.

Physical Examination

The first visit typically involves a physical examination. A thorough exam will involve checking the following:

- *Weight.* Find out whether your weight is within the normal range and ask for ways to lose weight, if necessary. Bringing your weight down to a healthy level can help you control blood sugar levels.
- *Blood pressure.* High blood pressure, which is generally anything above 140/90 mm/Hg, is a dangerous companion with diabetes. Both conditions are damaging to the blood vessels, and together, can increase your odds for developing heart attack or stroke. Be sure to find out what your reading says. Then ask your doctor for suggestions on how to lower your blood pressure.

- *Eye exam.* Although a specialist can provide a more detailed exam, a primary care doctor can usually alert you to signs of potential problems.
- *Feet.* Your doctor will do an exam of your feet by checking for any breaks that could lead to an infection and any signs of poor circulation, such as swelling, coldness, shiny skin, or thickened toe nails. Your doctor may also examine your feet for deformities such as calluses, corns, and ulcers, which indicate the need for better-fitting shoes.
- *Skin.* Diabetics are prone to bacterial and fungal infections on the skin. An examination of your entire body by your doctor can help detect those problems. Sometimes, a skin problem, such as a rash or hives, is a reaction to medication or insulin.
- *Mouth.* Your doctor will look inside your mouth for problems in your gums, teeth, mouth, and throat.

Blood and Urine Tests
On your first and subsequent visits, you will most likely be asked to provide a sample of your blood and urine. These body fluids provide a wealth of information and offer a glimpse into your health that cannot be detected otherwise.

Blood Tests
A laboratory analysis of your blood will reveal:
- *Blood glucose levels.*
- *Glycated hemoglobin levels, known as the HbA1C test.* This test, which some experts call the test with a memory, reveals how well you've been maintaining your blood glucose levels over the last two or three months. It gives you a bigger picture of how well you are controlling your blood glucose levels.

  Once the sample is retrieved, hemoglobin molecules in red blood cells are checked to see if they are glycated, or coated in sugar. The more glucose you have in your blood, the more glycated hemoglobin you will have. Healthy people usually have a 5 percent reading. Diabetics should strive for a reading of 7 percent or less. At that level, you are less likely to develop eye, kidney, and nerve disease than if the reading were higher.

- *Lipid profile, or cholesterol test.* A lipid profile will tell you how much cholesterol is circulating in your blood. High levels of total cholesterol are linked to cardiovascular disease, and especially dangerous for diabetics. In addition, a lipid profile reveals levels of low-density lipoproteins (LDLs), considered the "bad cholesterol" and high-density lipoproteins (HDLs), known as the "good cholesterol." It also provides information about your triglycerides, the most common form of stored fat in your body. High levels of triglycerides have been linked to cardiovascular disease.
- *Serum creatinine concentrations.* High levels of creatinine are an indication of a decline in kidney function.

Urine Test
A sample of your urine also provides a lot of information, including:

- *Ketones.* Poorly managed glucose levels may result in ketones in the urine, which are produced when the body is breaking down fats for energy. Too many ketones may indicate diabetic ketoacidosis, a potentially fatal condition brought on by inadequate amounts of insulin in the blood.
- *Protein.* High levels of certain proteins in your urine may suggest you are developing kidney disease. Impaired kidneys fail to separate a protein called albumin from the blood, and instead allow it to leak into the urine, causing a condition called microalbuminuria. If large quantities are present, it is called macroalbuminuria. It is commonly associated with hypertension. Blood

pressure medications can protect the kidneys and prevent or delay the complications. Left untreated, microalbuminuria can eventually lead to end-stage renal disease in which your kidneys no longer function without dialysis or a transplant.

How Often Should I See My Medical Team?

The frequency of your doctor visits will depend on your health and how well you're managing your blood glucose levels. If you're able to keep blood glucose levels in a healthy range, and you feel well, then you don't need to see your doctor more than once every three months. These routine checkups provide a great opportunity to assess just how well you're doing, and determine whether you're meeting goals such as losing weight or lowering your blood pressure. It's also a chance to simply talk about living with the disease.

However, if you're having trouble keeping blood glucose levels down, or you notice other symptoms, you may need to see your doctor or a specialist on your team more often. If you're starting a new medication, changing the dose of your medication or unable to get your blood glucose levels under control, you may need to see your doctor as often as every day for a while until your blood glucose levels stabilize.

Below is a medical to-do list for general diabetes care, provided by the American Diabetes Association:

Every three to six months:
  • Dental visit.
  • The A1C test.

Every year:
  • Get a blood test that checks cholesterol and serum creatinine levels.
  • Have your urine tested for infection, ketones, and protein levels.
  • Have an eye exam done by an ophthalmologist or optometrist.

- Get a flu shot.
- Visit your dietitian to review your meal plan and make sure it still satisfies your needs.
- Consult with your diabetes educator and provide an update of your health status.

Affordable Health Care

As everyone knows, medical care is very expensive these days. For people with diabetes, the costs can become quite high, with doctor visits, medications, and blood glucose monitoring supplies. A person with diabetes spent an average of $13,243 in 2002, compared with a healthy person whose health care expenses totaled $2,560.

That's why health insurance is absolutely essential for the person who has diabetes. You don't want financial constraints to ever affect the care you receive. And you don't need to cope with the stress of monetary concerns on top of managing your disease.

Whether you have a plan through your employer, an individual plan, or Medicare or Medicaid, make sure to do your research and find out what is covered in your diabetes care. Coverage can vary widely from one insurance plan to the next, and you want to make sure that yours is adequate for your health care and financial situation.

Below is a list of questions from the American Diabetes Association that you should answer about your health insurance coverage. Use these as a guide to help you compare your insurance options:

- Does the plan cover visits to your primary care physician? How many visits are you allowed? Is there a copayment involved?
- Does the plan reimburse you for diabetes education?
- Does the plan cover the cost of medical equipment and supplies, such as a blood glucose monitor or insulin?
- Will the plan cover consultations with a dietitian?
- What kind of coverage can you get for mental health services you might need?

- Does the plan cover the services of specialists, such as a podiatrist, eye doctor, or dentist?
- Does the plan cover the medications involved? Is there a prescription plan to help lower those costs? What are the copayments, if any?
- What kind of home health-care coverage does the plan provide?

CHAPTER THREE

Getting Blood Glucose Under Control

For years, you probably never gave much thought to your blood glucose levels. Maybe you didn't even know you had sugar in your blood or what it did in your body. But now that you have diabetes, you will give a lot more thought to it.

Because your body no longer regulates blood glucose levels in the normal range, that task now falls upon you. It won't be an easy job at first because blood glucose levels are highly sensitive and can swing wildly, depending on what you eat, how much you exercise and the kinds of medications you're taking. A simple cold can upset your blood glucose levels. So can a fight with your boss or a bad traffic jam.

Between finger sticks and keeping a logbook, you may consider it a nuisance to test your blood sugars. But keeping track of your blood sugar is vital to your health as a diabetic. The information you derive from monitoring your glucose will help you orchestrate the balancing of your insulin, medications, diet, and activity levels. All this might sound like a lot of work, but getting your blood glucose under control is the key to controlling your diabetes and keeping complications at bay. It will be as essential to your health and well-being as taking your medication, sticking to a balanced diet, and getting regular exercise.

Who Needs to Self-Monitor

Different people have different needs when it comes to monitoring blood glucose, but everyone has the same goal: to keep blood glucose levels as close to normal as possible. A normal blood sugar is usually maintained between 60 and 100 mg/dl. It's especially important for people with Type 1 diabetes or diabetics who rely on insulin or oral medications to keep track of their blood glucose levels. Regular monitoring will tell you how effectively your medications are working, and whether you need to increase or decrease the dosage. It can also tell you how your exercise habits are affecting blood glucose and whether that might impact your medication. In addition, it can help you detect a potentially dangerous bout of low blood sugar, which is always a risk if you are on medications.

People who have Type 2 diabetes and don't use medications or insulin don't need to monitor as frequently. But they can still benefit from keeping tabs on their blood glucose. Routine checks can help you see the impact of your diet and exercise. It may confirm that regular activity really does help lower your blood glucose levels or show you the effects that different foods have on your blood glucose.

Healthy Reasons to Self-Monitor

Self-monitoring of blood glucose is a relatively new phenomenon. Until the 1970s, patients relied on their doctors to determine blood glucose levels. But in 1971, the first blood glucose meter was patented. A diabetic physician named Richard K. Bernstein, who was insulin-dependent, wrote about his experiences with self-monitoring and published his findings in a book, *Dr. Bernstein's Diabetes Solution: A Complete Guide to Achieving Normal Blood Sugars.*

Over the years, more evidence began to reveal the effectiveness of self-monitoring. In 1986, the American Diabetes Association, the Centers for Disease Control and Prevention, the Food and Drug Administration, and the National Institutes of Health concluded that self-monitoring of blood glucose (SMBG) was an effective tool for diabetics that could help them make daily decisions on blood glucose control and recognize emergency situations. It was also an effective way to help patients track glucose levels over time and learn more about their condition. Better glucose control, it was thought, would help reduce the likelihood of complications and improve health.

In 1983, the National Institute of Diabetes and Digestive and Kidney Diseases (NIDDK) began its famous Diabetes Control and Complications Trial. The study involved patients from twenty-nine medical centers in the United States and Canada and set out to determine whether keeping blood glucose levels as close to normal as possible would lower the risk for complications.

The 1,441 people in the study were divided into two groups. One group followed standard treatment protocol. The conventional treatment group continued the same or similar dose of insulin at the same times each day, usually in the morning and evening, and checking glucose levels two or three times a day using a urine or blood test. The intensive treatment group injected insulin three or four times a day, self-monitoring blood glucose four to seven times a day, and adjusting insulin to food intake and activity levels.

The results were outstanding and showed the tremendous effect that intensive treatment could have on the disease. After ten years, patients who had practiced the intensive form of therapy were able to reduce their risk for retinopathy, or diabetic eye disease by 76 percent. Even patients who had early signs of retinopathy at the start of the study were able to slow the progression of the disease by 54 percent. The intensive group also was able to lower their odds of developing high cholesterol by 35 percent, nerve disease by 60 percent, and kidney disease by 50 percent.

Today, self-monitoring is regarded as a critical part of any diabetes treatment plan. To patients just beginning to understand the disease, it might seem overwhelming. But monitoring does get easier with practice and remains a vital part of your care. Only by monitoring your blood sugar are you able to know whether your treatment plan is working. You will also develop a better understanding of what specifically affects your blood glucose, how you might be able to impact it, and most important, how you can bring it back to healthy levels.

Glucose Basics

Glucose is a sugar derived primarily from the food you eat. Starches and other carbohydrates have a bigger influence on blood sugar after meals. Once digested, the sugar (glucose) travels into the bloodstream, where the hormone insulin lets it into body cells for conversion into energy. In people who have diabetes, the insulin-sensitive liver, muscle, and fat cells don't respond to the insulin or the body doesn't produce enough insulin. The result? The glucose lingers in the bloodstream until it's excreted in urine or metabolized by other tissues. In the meantime, it can cause extensive damage throughout the body if left untreated.

For people with diabetes, getting the amount of glucose in your blood to a normal level can be a challenge. Sometimes blood glucose levels can fall, causing "hypoglycemia" or low blood glucose. Other times, the levels can go too high, and set off a bout of "hyperglycemia" or high blood glucose.

Avoiding these excessive highs and lows takes practice and a constant balancing of food intake, exercise, medications, and insulin. It helps to understand how these factors impact your blood sugar levels.

Food

Okay, you slipped and went on an eating binge at the company's holiday party. Or maybe you couldn't eat lunch during a job interview because of a bad case of the jitters. Either way, you've disrupted your blood glucose levels, and your body is going to react, either by having too much glucose, as in the example of the party, or too little glucose, as in the case of the missed meal.

The food you eat can make a big difference in your blood glucose. The impact depends on how many carbohydrates are in a food, whether it's a sugar or a starch, and whether you ate it with something else. A potato for instance, contains more carbohydrates than a high-protein food such as pork, and will release more glucose. Simple sugars like fruit juice release glucose quickly, while starches like whole-wheat rice will do it more slowly. But if you drink the fruit juice with something that contains fat, such as ice cream, you'll slow down the action of glucose. That's because foods with protein and fat are digested more slowly than carbohydrates. Fats in the diet cause the intestine to secrete a hormone called "cholecystokinin," that delays the emptying of the stomach and allows the carbohydrates to be absorbed more slowly. High fiber foods can have a similar effect on delaying the absorption of carbohydrates.

The amount you eat also matters. Eating too much can send blood glucose levels upward, while not eating enough can cause them to plummet.

Exercise

If you've noticed that your blood glucose levels are closer to normal after a long walk, then you've already seen the effects that physical activity can have on blood glucose. Exercise uses up the glucose circulating in your blood. During a workout, your muscles burn up glucose. When those stores are exhausted, your body taps into blood glucose to keep you going. Exercise also makes muscles and tissues more sensitive to the effects of insulin. In general, the more active you are, the lower your blood glucose.

Strenuous exercise may have an effect on your blood sugar for up to twelve hours after the activity. Therefore, exercise in the evening hours may cause the blood glucose to drop during the night, especially if you are on insulin, a condition known as nocturnal hypoglycemia. Monitoring at bedtime is important to ensure the blood glucose is high enough, and a bedtime snack may be needed to prevent the nighttime drop in blood glucose.

Insulin and Oral Diabetes Medications

If you use insulin or medications to treat your diabetes, you're vulnerable to changes in your blood sugar. Both treatments work to lower blood glucose levels, but they can be greatly affected by the time they're administered and the type of food you eat.

If you don't time your insulin injection or medications correctly, your blood glucose can swing high or low. For instance, if you eat right after an injection, the insulin won't be effective yet, and blood glucose can climb too high. Wait too long, and the levels can go too low.

The amount you eat can affect the impact of your insulin or medication, too. Eating more than you planned can give you a bout of high blood glucose. There won't be enough insulin or medication in your body to handle the extra sugar. On the other hand, if you eat less than you had planned, you'll wind up with low blood sugar.

Illness

Being sick causes stress on the body. In response, the release of counter regulatory hormones—including cortisone, adrenaline, growth hormone, and glucagon—will automatically increase blood glucose levels. The extra sugar helps the body recover, but in people who have diabetes, the process may work against the effects of insulin and result in hyperglycemia. During an illness, you'll need to monitor your blood glucose more frequently. As a result, you may need to make adjustments to your diet, insulin, and medications to account for the fluctuation. You may also need to keep closer watch over ketone levels in your urine.

Stress

A bad day at the office. An impending deadline. A fight with your spouse. All these stressors release a cocktail of hormones that can push blood glucose up. If you're feeling stressed, your glucose levels may be higher than usual.

Measuring Blood Glucose

Getting a reading of your blood glucose level is actually a quick two-minute process. But to do it, you'll need some special equipment.

- *Lancet.* A lancet is a small sharp device that draws blood with a quick stick of the finger or forearm. There are several kinds of lancets on the market, but try to find one that delivers the shallowest poke to reduce pain and scarring. Some lancets are attached to a lancing device, called an automatic lancet device. These are the easiest to use, draw the most consistent amounts of blood and can be easily used to obtain a sample of blood from either hand. But when you buy an automatic lancet device, you'll need to buy the actual lancets separately, which can get expensive. Lancets may be used over again by one person on several occasions if they are wiped off with alcohol after each use. But keep in mind that different lancets produce different sized drops of blood. Make sure to use one that gets a large enough drop of blood to cover a test strip.
- *Test strips.* After you draw the blood, you'll wipe it on a test strip that's been chemically treated to test for glucose. When the blood touches the test strip, the color of the test strip changes. The strip is then inserted into the monitor, which then reads it and tells you how much glucose is present.
- *Blood glucose monitor, or meter.* The monitor or meter is a computerized device that reads information about your blood glucose from the test strip. Some monitors measure a color assay, while others measure an electric current. Some fancier models now even measure both blood glucose and glycated hemoglobin, and blood glucose and ketones. Another monitor goes so far as

to measure blood glucose, ketones, and lipids, including cholesterol, triglycerides, and HDL. Choosing the right monitor will depend on several factors, which we'll discuss later.

- *Journal or log book.* Sure, you'll need to know your blood glucose before a meal or after you exercise. But only by keeping track of your levels over a period of time can you get a better idea of what affects your blood glucose and how you can keep it under control. Each time you check your blood glucose, record the date and time, the test result, and the type and dosage of any medication you're taking. You might also note any special circumstances such as a change in the most recent meal, activity levels, or overall health. Most meters come with a log book, but you can also get one from your diabetes educator or physician. You should have space to record the time, date and blood glucose, as well as any special circumstances or comments about your health.

If you prefer to go high-tech, consider purchasing a data management system, which measures your blood glucose and also stores information about date, time, reading, insulin, exercise, and diet. Some systems will allow you to download the information onto your computer or your doctor's computer. Other fancier versions will even provide a complete analysis of your data.

When to Check

How frequently you check your blood glucose varies, depending on whether you take insulin and how well your blood sugar is controlled. In general, if you're taking insulin, it's a good idea to check before every meal or big snack, and again one to two hours after you eat. You should also check before bed and once in the middle of the night to make sure it's not dipping too low.

If you were recently diagnosed with diabetes, you may also test more frequently in order to detect patterns in your blood glucose. And according to the American Diabetes Association, it's also a good idea to do more frequent checks if you:

- Are sick.
- Suspect low blood glucose.
- Are pregnant or considering getting pregnant.
- Have been experiencing fluctuations in blood glucose that are extremely high or low.
- Recently gained or lost weight.
- Just started taking a non-diabetes or over-the-counter drug that could affect blood glucose or your ability to spot the signs of low blood glucose.
- Are changing your exercise, diet, insulin, or medications.
- Are about to drive, and you take insulin or sulfonylureas.
- Are about to engage in physical activity.
- Suffer from frequent insulin reactions overnight or wake up with very high blood glucose.
- Have trouble recognizing symptoms of low blood glucose.
- Are on intensive insulin therapy.

Selecting a Monitor

Choosing a blood glucose monitor is a bit like choosing a car. There are several makes and models, each with its own features. Only you can decide which monitor works best.

Work with your diabetes educator or primary care doctor to determine the right model for you. Some things you might want to consider:

- Is the monitor the right size for you?
- Is this monitor affordable?
- Is the device easy to maintain, clean, and operate?
- Can I read the monitor easily?

- Do I want a monitor with memory?
- Can I get a big enough drop of blood to satisfy the strips used in my monitor?
- How often do I need to calibrate the monitor?
- How often does it need new batteries?
- Does my insurance plan cover the meter or the test strips?

Other Ways to Measure Blood Glucose

Scientists have been researching noninvasive methods of measuring blood glucose, which do not require puncturing the skin. These methods are not designed to replace blood glucose monitors, but rather to act as a supplement that provides additional information about patterns in your blood glucose levels.

Among the first of these devices to hit the market was the Gluco-Watch Biographer, made by Cygnus, Inc. The device is worn like a watch on the wrist and uses a sensor to detect blood glucose levels in perspiration. The watch is calibrated in the morning and worn throughout the day. Readings are given every twenty minutes.

But the watch is far from ideal. The watch is expensive to use, and you still need regular glucose monitoring to set it. Also, the pad is good for only twelve hours, and then a new pad must be applied. Irritation at the site frequently occurs and prevents future use of the watch. In addition, it takes three hours for the pad to achieve equilibrium, so it is used effectively for only nine of the twelve hours.

Researchers are continuing to experiment with other noninvasive methods for measuring blood glucose. One technology uses a beam of light on the skin to read glucose levels. Another system, called the Mini-Med Continuous Glucose Monitoring System, uses a small catheter inserted just below the skin. The catheter collects liquid that is then passed through a biosensor. The MiniMed is not designed for daily blood glucose checks, but rather for periodic usage and for identifying trends in blood glucose levels.

Some glucose monitors are designed to test blood from alternative sites on the body. The preferred site for measuring blood glucose is in the fingertips, where changes in glucose levels turn up more quickly than elsewhere on the body. Alternative sites for testing include the upper arm, forearm, base of the thumb, and thigh.

Under regulations by the U.S. Food and Drug Administration, devices that allow for alternative site testing must clearly show that there are no differences between blood testing at these alternative locations and fingertips. But if there are possible differences, the manufacturer must inform consumers about times when blood glucose is most prone to change—after a meal, taking insulin, or after exercising. They must also suggest fingertip sampling if the patient suspects low blood sugar, is unable to detect signs of hypoglycemia, or test results don't agree with how the patient feels.

Accuracy Concerns

Perhaps you're a neophyte in the monitoring process. Or maybe you bought a package of generic test strips that didn't quite fit in your monitor. Or perhaps you just handled something sweet like an apple before you put your blood onto the test strip.

Like any process, monitoring your blood glucose can be highly imperfect, causing results to be higher or lower than they actually are. Most errors are human ones that can be easily corrected. Some are related to the equipment you're using. Below are some common situations that can alter the accuracy of your reading:

- Your meter is dirty or damaged.
- The test strips you're using don't work with your meter.
- The test strips are expired or damaged.
- The batteries in your meter need replacement.
- You didn't get enough blood on the test strip.
- You got too much blood on the test strip.

- The meter was not at room temperature.
- The meter recently experienced a change of altitude or humidity.
- You have a health condition that affects hematocrit, the amount of red blood cells in your blood. Low levels of hematocrit usually test higher for blood glucose. High levels of hematocrit usually test lower for blood glucose.
- Your fingertips were dirty or sticky when you withdrew blood.

Check Your Meter for Accuracy

There are essentially two ways you can make sure your monitor is working up to par. One way is to test quality control solutions or electronic controls to measure the accuracy of your monitor. These tests use a liquid control solution instead of your blood. The solution contains a known amount of glucose, so you know what the result of a reading should be. With an electronic control, you place a cartridge or special "control" test strip in the meter. A signal will indicate whether your meter works.

Another way to ensure your meter is working for you is to take it to the doctor's office. Demonstrate for your doctor how you use it, so he can point out any mistakes in your procedure. Your doctor can also do a blood glucose check and compare the values obtained from a laboratory against those from your meter. If the results do not match, you may need to consider getting a new monitor.

What's Normal Anyway?

Now that you know how to do a glucose check, you need to determine where you want your blood glucose to be. The American Diabetes Association suggests the following goals:

Before meals: Persons without diabetes should usually have readings of 110 mg/dl or lower. Diabetics should aim for 80 to 120 mg/dl.

Before bedtime: Healthy people usually have readings of less than 120 mg/dl. Diabetics should aim for readings of 100 to 140 mg/dl.

Some of these numbers might seem unrealistic or unattainable to you. Keep in mind though, that everyone will have different goals, depending on your age, your health, and your ability to recognize symptoms of low blood sugar. If you're older, your health may be compromised by complications from diabetes, and your goals may be higher. Younger adults who can easily spot the signs of low blood sugar may have goals closer to those recommended by the ADA. Children might have slightly lower goals. Pinpointing your goals will require working closely with your primary care doctor.

When Blood Glucose Levels Are Low

Blood glucose readings that are lower than normal indicate you might be at risk for hypoglycemia or low blood sugar. The condition is most common in people who have Type 1 diabetes and other diabetics who rely on insulin or sulfonylurea drugs to lower their glucose. Once insulin or drugs are in the body, there is nothing to stop these treatments from working and doing their job of removing blood glucose. But sometimes, they simply do it too well. Left untreated, hypoglycemia can lead to unconsciousness.

Some people know they're having a bout of hypoglycemia even before they check their blood glucose. They might feel shaky, weak, dizzy, or faint. You might also have difficulty concentrating and feel nervous, hungry, and irritable.

But some patients may have no idea that their blood glucose levels are falling, a condition known as hypoglycemia unawareness. Pregnant women are vulnerable to hypoglycemia unawareness as are people whose first sign of low blood sugar is impaired thinking. The best way to handle it is to prevent even mild levels of hypoglycemia by doing more frequent blood glucose checks, testing every time before you drive, and alerting the people around you that you are prone to this problem.

What to do: If your blood glucose is low, you need to eat a fast-acting carbohydrate. Wait fifteen minutes, and then test it again. If your reaction is severe, you will need to seek emergency medical treatment.

If you planned ahead, you may have gotten a prescription for a glucagon kit. A family member or friend should be trained to use it. Glucagon is injected intramuscularly and causes the liver to release glycogen, which is glucose stored in the liver. With glucagon, blood glucose increases rapidly in five to ten minutes, and may prevent a seizure and the need to call 911 and an ambulance.

When Blood Glucose Levels Are High

A blood glucose reading that is too high is a sign of hyperglycemia, or high blood sugar. If your blood glucose is chronically high, you may develop complications of diabetes.

Signs of hyperglycemia are often subtle. You may feel thirstier than usual and have a stronger than normal urge to urinate. You may also feel fatigued or have blurry vision.

In people who have Type 1 diabetes, high blood glucose can lead to diabetic ketoacidosis or DKA, a rare condition caused by inadequate amounts of insulin. Without enough insulin, your liver gets the signal to break down fat for energy. The process produces ketones, toxic acids that can build up in the blood, causing DKA, which can lead to coma and death.

The risk for people with Type 2 diabetes is hyperglycemic hyperosmolar non-ketotic coma, or HHNC, a condition that commonly occurs among the elderly. To eliminate the excess glucose, your body produces more urine, causing your body to dehydrate. The process may last for several days, and a state of extreme confusion may occur, so that you are unable to get even a drink of water. Like DKA, if HHNC goes untreated, you may experience coma and death.

What to do: If your blood glucose is above 350 mg/dl, you should call a member of your medical team immediately. You may require a fast-acting insulin. Drink water to prevent dehydrating, and avoid exercise, which can further raise blood glucose.

If you suspect DKA and your blood glucose is over 250 mg/dl, call a member of your health team. Do a urine test for ketones. If you think you might have HHS, and blood glucose is above 350 mg/dl, call someone on your health team right away. If your blood glucose is over 500 mg/dl, get to an emergency room immediately.

A Final Note

Like anything, monitoring your glucose is something that will become easier with practice. The finger pricks of a lancet will become less painful. The signs of hypoglycemia will become more obvious. And you'll become accustomed to pausing for a blood glucose check before you eat a meal.

Monitoring blood glucose is among the most important things a diabetic can do to take care of her health and avoid the complications of the disease. So even if you never become accustomed to the finger pricks and still find the checks a nuisance, don't ever give up the practice. New, less invasive devices are under development, including a patch that can draw glucose from the fluids in your skin and the use of near infrared light beams that detect the presence of blood sugar in skin tissue. In the meantime, work with your medical team to find a monitor that suits your financial situation, lifestyle, needs, and schedule. Your efforts will be well worth it.

A PERSONAL STORY

Bill

Bill was forty-eight when the doctor told him he had diabetes. Except for high blood pressure, he'd always been fairly healthy. But a couple of years ago, Bill noticed he was drinking more than usual. Nothing seemed to satisfy his thirst. He was also going to the bathroom more frequently and feeling unusually tired. At first, he attributed these symptoms to the stress of his job as an engineer. But just to be safe, Bill went to the doctor.

The doctor's news was grim: Not only did Bill have elevated blood glucose levels, but he also had high blood pressure and high cholesterol. He was also twenty pounds overweight.

"I think I'd taken my good health for granted," Bill says. "It wasn't as if I was super heavy or unable to move around. But the triple whammy scared me."

Bill was told to start by trying to lose weight with diet and exercise. The lifestyle change was a struggle, he admits, because he never had to diet before. He had always eaten a meat and potatoes diet, not one laden with fruits and vegetables. He also wasn't a fan of exercise. A former high school baseball player and avid golfer, Bill liked activities, but hated the idea of exercise alone.

"My wife really started getting on my case to eat better, and she started cooking healthier meals," Bill says. "She bought all these cookbooks with low-fat recipes and started buying more fruits and vegetables. She also cleared the cabinets of all my favorite treats, like Oreos, nacho chips, and other bad snacks. Looking back, I think she probably saved my life."

The couple also began taking nightly walks after dinner. Sometimes, they walked a mile through the neighborhood. Other times, they went on two-mile treks through town. Though Bill initially balked at the idea of walking every night, he grew to enjoy these outings.

In two months, Bill shed ten pounds. He felt more energetic and was sleeping better. For Christmas, his wife bought him a blood glucose monitor and blood pressure monitor to help him check his own numbers. Both numbers had improved since his visit to the doctor.

The next time he went to see his doctor, he was congratulated on all the progress he'd made. But Bill's blood glucose numbers were still slightly elevated, and his doctor put him on Glucophage to help make sure the weight didn't come back. "I really didn't want to take any medication, because I didn't like knowing I had diabetes," Bill says. "I had done some reading and knew about the complications of the disease. It was not a pretty picture, and to be honest, I was frightened."

The medication did the trick. In a few months, Bill's blood glucose levels were within the normal range. The doctor let him stop the Glucophage and rely instead just on diet and exercise for managing his blood sugars. The lifestyle changes also made an impact on his blood pressure and cholesterol, which have both fallen since he lost the extra weight. "But occasionally, when I'm under a lot of stress, I know my blood pressure can go high," he says. "I try to lower it by walking a little extra and eating less salt."

So far so good. Bill, now fifty, is pleased knowing that he was able to take control of his health and hopes he can continue to do so. "The last thing I want is to spend my retirement years dealing with complications from diabetes," he says. "I have other things I'd rather do, like golfing and hiking."

CHAPTER FOUR

Diet and Exercise

All your life, you ate pretty much whatever you wanted. Maybe you enjoyed Friday night pizza parties, indulged in your share of sweets, and frequented all-you-can-eat buffets, never thinking twice about that second helping of mashed potatoes. Exercise? You did that when you could find the time. Maybe you visited the gym during the winter months, or exercised on the weekends. But most days, you were too busy to squeeze in any physical activity, so you put it off for another day.

Now that you've been diagnosed with diabetes, eating well and getting regular exercise can no longer be postponed. For a diabetic, smart eating and regular exercise are essential to controlling the disease and preventing future complications.

To do that, you will need to devise an individualized meal plan that suits your lifestyle and look for ways to incorporate exercise into your life. Good diet and exercise habits can make all the difference in how stable your blood glucose levels are and how well you can keep other complications from developing. Exercise and caloric restriction can help prevent the weight gain that can make diabetes so deadly, and also reduce your need for insulin.

Ideally, you'll seek out a dietitian to help you devise a customized eating plan that suits your lifestyle. And perhaps you'll enlist the aid of an exercise physiologist or a trainer at a health club for assistance in creating a fitness plan. But in the meantime, it helps to have a basic understanding of why diet and exercise play such a major role in diabetes management.

The Nutrition Basics

Paying close attention to what you eat is an important part of regulating your blood glucose, so it helps to understand how different nutrients affect your health and well-being. But first, you need to know what they are.

Carbohydrates

Carbohydrates are your body's primary source of energy and come in two forms of sugars: simple and complex. Simple carbohydrates are found naturally in fruits, vegetables, and milk, but are also in foods that contain refined sugars, which have been processed to extract the natural sucrose found in plants to sweeten the flavor. Nutritionally, refined sugars are considered empty calories, foods that provide energy but no vitamins or minerals. Simple carbohydrates break down relatively quickly, causing blood sugars to rise more rapidly.

Complex carbohydrates are starches and fiber that are found in legumes, grains, and vegetables. Starch is derived from the storage systems of plants, such as beans, lentils, potatoes, wheat, or oats. Like the sugars found in simple carbohydrates, starches break down into simple sugars, but do so more slowly.

Fiber, on the other hand, cannot be digested in the stomach at all because humans lack the enzymes to break it down. There are two kinds of fiber:

- Soluble fibers can dissolve in water and are found in dried peas and beans, apples, carrots, and oats. Soluble fibers are especially important to diabetics because they lower the levels of blood sugar and reduce the need for insulin or medication. Although the reasons are not clearly understood, soluble fiber reduces the time it takes to empty the stomach, which in turn delays the absorption of glucose into the bloodstream and lowers the need for insulin. Soluble fibers also help reduce cholesterol levels. The fibers bind to bile acids, which are made of cholesterol, and transport them out of the body as waste.

• Insoluble fibers, also called roughage, do not dissolve in water and are found in whole-wheat foods, green beans, wheat bran, and broccoli. Because insoluble fibers absorb water, they can add bulk to the stool and help move food through the digestive tract more quickly.

Protein

Athletes training for major events are often told to eat protein to build muscle. That's because proteins supply the amino acids that help the body build, repair, and maintain body tissues. You can find protein in meats, eggs, legumes, nuts, seeds, soybeans, and tofu. In the absence of carbohydrates, excess protein may be used for energy.

Diabetics need to be wary of high-protein diets, especially if they have kidney disease. Too much protein can tax the kidneys and promote kidney failure. Diabetics should limit protein intake to no more than sixty to eighty grams per day. In people who have kidney disease, it is often limited to less than forty grams per day. Too much protein in your diet can also promote weight gain since most high-protein foods are also high in saturated fat and cholesterol. Any excess protein is stored as fat.

A healthier way to satisfy your protein needs would be to consume more plant foods, such as beans, chickpeas, broccoli, and spinach. These foods also supply other nutrients, including fiber and essential vitamins.

Fats

When you dive into a bowl of ice cream, the substance that gives it its wonderful, creamy texture is fat. That's the same stuff that makes a cinnamon bun so tasty and a slice of cheesecake so delectable. But too much of it can be unhealthy and fattening.

Fats are organic compounds that play a critical role in the brain and nervous system. They are also the most concentrated source of energy, providing nine calories per gram, compared with four calories per gram for carbohydrates or protein. Too much fat of any kind can cause weight gain, which is especially unhealthy for diabetics.

Fats come in two basic forms, saturated and unsaturated. Saturated fats, which are unhealthy fats, are solid at room temperature and come from meat, whole dairy products, butter, and palm and coconut oils. A diet rich in saturated fats can clog arteries and raise your risk for heart disease.

Unsaturated fats are the healthier fats and come in two forms. The monounsaturated variety comes from nuts, avocados, and olive oil. Polyunsaturated fats are liquids found mostly in vegetable oils, such as safflower, sunflower, and corn. They are also found in fish in the form of omega-3 fatty acids.

Another type of fat that has gotten a great deal of notoriety is trans fatty acids, which are formed when oils are hydrogenated to make them solid at room temperature. In foods, hydrogenation helps enhance the shelf life of processed foods.

Trans fatty acids are getting a lot of publicity these days because of their connection to high cholesterol and heart disease. Unfortunately, it's hard to escape these fatty acids. Hydrogenated and partially hydrogenated oils are used in all kinds of processed foods, including breakfast cereals, frozen waffles, granola bars, potato chips, cookies, crackers, and more. It's also in margarine and shortening. Fortunately, new food labels will reveal the content of trans fatty acids in these foods, so consumers can make smarter choices.

Fat can impact blood glucose levels by promoting weight gain, which makes your body more resistant to insulin. Fat also slows the absorption of carbohydrates, which your body needs for energy. That means that if you eat a lot of fat and carbs together (pizza is a classic example), your blood sugar will take longer to rise than if you had the same amount of carbs alone. The delay may affect the amount of insulin you need before that meal.

Cholesterol

Our bodies manufacture cholesterol, a waxy fat-like substance that is vital to making and repairing cell membranes, and producing important hormones such as estrogen and testosterone. You can also get cholesterol from foods such as meat, butter, and cheese.

Too much cholesterol in your diet can raise total blood cholesterol levels, which increases your risk for atherosclerosis, a disease characterized by hardening of the arteries, and heart disease. But it's also important to have low levels of LDLs, or low-density lipoproteins. Dubbed the "bad or harmful cholesterol," LDLs are responsible for bringing cholesterol throughout the body, where they can build up on blood vessel walls. Eventually, a plaque forms, causing the arteries to harden and narrow.

On the other hand, you do want high levels of HDLs, or high-density lipoproteins. The HDLs are known as "the good cholesterol" that scoop up excess cholesterol and bring it to the liver, where it is broken down and eliminated.

The Sweet Stuff

In the old days, diabetics were urged to steer clear of all sweets. Sugar, it was believed, was the biggest culprit behind the disease. So it was acceptable to eat potatoes, rice, and pasta, but you were supposed to stay away from cake, cookies, and ice cream.

It turns out that sugar got a bad rap. Whether it's the sucrose in an orange or the starch in corn, the rate that blood glucose levels rise is the same, no matter what the source of the carbohydrate. That means that even the occasional sweet can still be a part of a healthy diabetic diet.

The problem with most sugary foods is that they contain refined sugars, which are void of nutritional benefits, or what dietitians call empty calories. In fact, many of these foods are often high in calories, which can make weight gain more problematic. So before you indulge in too many sweets, be sure you aren't enjoying them at the expense of other more nutrient-rich foods that are less likely to add inches to your waistline.

Putting It All Together

Changing the way you eat may seem like a daunting feat. You may still be reeling from the news that you have diabetes, and trying to make sense of the disease. To give up favorite dietary staples at this stressful time might simply seem too overwhelming. But the sooner you learn to eat a healthy diet, the more likely you are to get a handle on your blood glucose levels and prevent the harmful effects of diabetes.

Eating for diabetes is not unlike following a healthy, balanced diet. In fact, the two are virtually identical. You want to minimize your intake of calories, fat, and refined sugars while getting most of your calories from healthy foods like fruit, vegetables, and whole grains. You also want to eat a varied diet, but limit your intake of salt and refined sugars. If you have diabetes, you simply have to become hypervigilant about your carbohydrate intake since carbs are your body's primary source of blood glucose.

The goal of a diabetic meal plan isn't to eliminate all the foods you enjoy or to impose a regimen of foods you dislike. Rather, working with a registered dietitian, your new meal plan should be designed to fit your lifestyle, schedule, and tastes. Here are some general tips that might help you achieve that goal:

- *Space out your meals.* The time between meals, usually four to five hours, will allow your pancreas to produce insulin, if it still does, and for insulin medications to work without confronting large amounts of sugar in your blood.

- *Consider eating breakfast or a mid-morning meal.* An early meal helps you feel full, so you don't gorge later on. It also helps keep blood glucose levels at more even levels.
- *Eat a consistent amount from one day to the next.* It's dull to eat the same meals every day, but keeping the amount the same— especially carbohydrates—will help you achieve better glucose control.
- *Avoid skipping meals.* Missing a meal puts you at risk for overeating when you finally do eat and can make weight control more difficult.
- *Try to eat at the same time everyday.* Maintaining a consistent eating schedule will help stabilize your blood sugar levels.

Carbohydrate Counting

The newest dietary strategy for managing diabetes is to count the carbohydrate content of every meal and snack, a method known as carb counting that gained popularity in the 1990s. Virtually all the glucose circulating in your blood after a meal comes from carbohydrates, which include everything from fruits, vegetables, and pasta to popcorn, cakes, and crackers.

Although carb counting can help anyone with diabetes, it is especially useful for people who rely on insulin or take a medication to manage their disease. Once you figure out how many carbs you're going to eat, you can adjust your insulin accordingly. Bolus insulin, the insulin you administer before or after a meal, works to reduce the glucose that comes primarily from carbohydrates. Basal insulin helps reduce the glucose that comes from proteins and fats, which take longer to be metabolized and broken down into glucose.

You can also adjust the amount of carbs you eat, depending on the blood glucose reading before the meal or snack. And if you want to eat more carbs than usual at a special meal, such as Thanksgiving, you can adjust your insulin accordingly.

On ordinary days however, the goal of carb counting is to simply keep the amount of carbs you eat consistent at each meal, every day. Eating the same amount at the same time every day allows for more stable blood glucose levels than if you were to eat random amounts throughout the day.

Counting Servings

One way to count carbs is to tally up your servings. Essentially, each serving of a starch, fruit, or milk has fifteen grams of carbohydrates. Vegetables have just five grams in a single serving. So if you eat three servings of a vegetable, you will have eaten the equivalent of a single starch, fruit, or milk.

To figure out what constitutes a serving, you should check the nutrition label. You can also find information about serving sizes in books published by the American Dietetic Association and the American Diabetes Association.

Counting carbs by servings is not an exact science, but an easier method of tracking your carb intake than adding up grams. After all, the fifteen grams per serving estimate is actually an average. In reality, one serving can contain as little as eleven grams of carbohydrates or as much as twenty. Because of the broad range, counting carbs by servings requires some judgment on your part. Do you need those few extra grams of carbs? Do you need the calories they'll add? And how will it affect your blood glucose levels if you eat those additional carbs?

Counting Grams

A more precise way to count carbs is to add up the grams in a serving of food. This method takes more effort, but is better suited to diabetics who prefer to be more accurate about their carb intake.

Say you want to eat thirty grams of carbohydrates at lunch. You would set out to create a meal that provides for that many carbs, usually with the goal of staying within five to seven grams. One slice of bread and an apple quickly add up to thirty grams. But so does a cup of soda and an oatmeal cookie. Of course, the first meal is the healthier option, even though the impact on blood glucose levels would be the same.

So if you do practice carb counting, keep in mind that the key is to plan a well-balanced meal with approximately 50 percent of calories coming from carbs. Resist the temptation to create a meal that focuses exclusively on one food group or overemphasizes sweets. Instead, make sure your carbohydrates always come from whole grains, fruits, and vegetables, and that sweets are kept to a minimum. Be sure the carbs are spread out evenly throughout the day at your meals.

Also, be wary of excessive snacking if you have Type 2 diabetes. Too many between-meal snacks can make it hard to lose weight. And the newer insulins, which are more predictable, can help prevent hypoglycemia without the use of snacks.

Purchase a carb counter book and write down everything you eat. Studies show that people who keep food diaries are more successful at weight maintenance.

The Exchange System

Before carb counting came into vogue, most diabetics were using the exchange system to organize their meals and snacks. The exchange system works by helping the patient eat a consistent amount of carbohydrates, protein, fat, and calories from day to day.

The system is organized into lists of six food groups, namely fruit, starch/bread, meat and meat substitutes, vegetables, fruit, milk, and fat. The foods on each list are similar to one another in terms of how many carbohydrates, protein, and fat they contain. They're also similar in terms of calorie content.

These similarities are achieved because each food on a list is assigned a serving size. For instance a small apple will share the list with half a cup of canned pears, which both contain fifteen grams of carbohydrates, sixty calories, and no fat. Also on the list are two tablespoons of raisins and a half cup of orange juice.

Working with a registered dietitian, you then devise a meal plan for each day that dictates how many servings should come from each category of food. For instance, at breakfast, you may have two servings of starch with one serving each of fruit, milk, meat, and fat. You then make your food choices based on which foods are on each list, making sure to satisfy your servings requirements. One day you may satisfy the breakfast milk requirements with one cup of 2 percent milk, the next with eight ounces of yogurt.

Like carb counting, the exchange system does allow flexibility in food choices. It's easy to exchange one food for another on the same list. But unlike carb counting, the exchange system incorporates meats, meat substitutes, and fats, which may help with overall meal planning.

What's the Glycemic Index?

Eat a slice of white bread, and your blood sugars are going to rise rapidly. But eat a bowl of ice cream, and the effect is a slow increase in blood glucose, thanks to the high fat content of ice cream.

The rate in which sugar is released into your bloodstream is the basis of another way to measure your food, called the glycemic index. The higher the index rating, the faster the food sends sugar into your blood. Food is measured against white bread or glucose, which is set at a value of 100 percent. Foods that raise glucose levels slower than white bread or glucose are rated below 100. Those include fruits, beans, and pasta. Some foods release sugars into the bloodstream faster than white bread does, including white bagels, cake, doughnuts, instant rice, and carrots.

The problem with the glycemic index is it is extremely imprecise. The glycemic index of any food varies greatly, depending on how the food was prepared, whether it was processed, and how it was served. Boiled potatoes for instance, have a lower glycemic index than instant potatoes. Less processed foods like fruits are usually lower on the glycemic index than refined foods. Even foods that appear the same can have different effects. For instance, skim milk has a more rapid effect on blood glucose than 2 percent milk. And if you eat a food that's high on the glycemic index with one that is low, you usually wind up lowering the glycemic index of the higher food. The glycemic index also varies with your diabetic medication, when you last took it, and the time you last ate.

So should you use the glycemic index to determine your meal plan? That depends. The index can be a valuable tool for assessing which foods affect your blood glucose levels. By testing your blood glucose levels after eating a particular food on several occasions, you might discover that the food tends to elevate blood sugar quickly. Perhaps you'll decide to shrink your serving size the next time or increase your medication.

But don't base your food choices entirely on the glycemic index. If you strive only to eat foods that are low on the index, you'll wind up omitting healthy options such as pasta and carrots or restricting your serving sizes of foods like fruit. Keep in mind that some foods that are low on the glycemic index have high amounts of other unhealthy nutrients. A good example is a candy bar, which contains a lot of saturated fat. Likewise, some foods low on the glycemic index are also healthy in other ways. Strawberries and other berries for instance, contain a lot of fiber and have a low glycemic index.

Remember that if a food is eaten alone as a snack, the glycemic index becomes more important because there are no other foods that can affect it. But when a food is eaten as part of a meal, the glycemic index becomes less important.

Useful Diet Tools

All this information is wasted if you don't use the right tools for creating a meal plan. Here are some helpful things you need to do to make your plan work for you.

Measure Your Portions

Many people who are overweight got there because their portion sizes were too large. They ordered super-sized servings in fast-food restaurants, devoured every bite of food on their plate long after they felt full, and gave in to the temptation to eat more.

Having diabetes means reducing those portions, so that your body is better able to tolerate the influx of sugar. More than ever, the amount you eat is just as important as what you eat.

The only way to know your portion is to measure what you eat, the same way you measure ingredients for a recipe. Keep your measuring tools—spoons, cups for both liquids and solids, and a food scale—handy. Practice measuring every morsel you eat, and placing the food on your plate. With practice, you'll develop an eye for gauging how much food you have in your bowl or plate. You may also discover that a tablespoon of peanut butter is not as much as you thought or that three ounces of chicken is really enough food for you.

Read Nutrition Labels

We're fortunate to live in an era when nutrition information is so readily available and literally at our fingertips. In 1994, the National Labeling Act went into effect, requiring food manufacturers to post nutrition labels on their products.

While shopping for your meal plan, always consult the information on the food label. The three components of a label are:

- *The nutrition facts panel.* By now, most of us are familiar with the box that outlines the content of carbs, protein, and fats we're eating. You can also find out how many calories are in a single serving as well as the sodium, sugar, and fiber content of that food. Most important perhaps, the panel reveals what constitutes a serving. Always check that information since a serving size may be much different from what you're accustomed to eating.

- *The ingredient list.* Printed on the side or back of the package, usually in smaller print, are the ingredients that go into producing the food. The ingredients are listed according to the amount in the food. So if sugar is the first ingredient, it means the food contains more sugar than the other ingredients listed after it. You can also find out whether the manufacturer used hydrogenated oils, artificial colors, preservatives, or sweeteners.

- *Nutrition claims.* These statements link the food to health concerns such as cholesterol, fat, sugar, and calories and are optional. Only health claims based on scientific research are allowed by the FDA. Each claim actually has very specific meanings attached to it. For instance calorie-free means the product has less than five calories per serving. If a product claims that sugar, fat, or calories are reduced, it usually means that there is 25 percent less of the substance than in the non-reduced version. A food that claims to be lowfat can have no more than three grams of fat in a serving.

What If I'm Counting Calories, Too?

Weight loss should be a goal for anyone who's carrying a few extra pounds, which could be as many as 90 percent of all diabetics. Even shedding a modest amount of weight, like ten to twenty pounds, can make a difference in blood glucose control and the amount of insulin and medications you might require. Losing weight is also accompanied by lower levels of LDL (the bad cholesterol), higher levels of HDL (the good cholesterol), lower triglycerides (derived from fats in foods and the liver), and lower blood pressure. Best of all, losing weight can improve your quality of life.

How do you know if you're overweight? That depends on your body mass index (BMI), a measure of weight for height in adults over twenty years old that correlates with body fat. You can find out your body mass index by checking out the website for the Centers for Disease Control and Prevention's National Center for Chronic Disease Prevention and Health Promotion at www.cdc.gov/nccdphp/dnpa/bmi/bmi-adult.htm

You can also calculate it yourself by using this formula: BMI= body weight in kilograms/height in meters x 2. To convert to the metric system, take your weight in pounds and divide it by 2.2 to determine your weight in kilograms. Next, divide your height in inches by 39.37 to determine your height in meters.

For example, if you weigh 200 pounds, and you are 5-foot 10-inches tall, you weigh 91 kg and are 1.78 meters tall. The formula for your BMI then is: BMI= 91/1.78 x 2 = 91/3.56 = 25.6.

If you have a body mass index of 25 to 29.9, you are considered overweight. Among adults aged 20 to 74, approximately 35 percent are overweight. Even more alarming are the growing numbers of people who are obese, which is defined as having a BMI greater than or equal to 30. Approximately 21 percent of American adults are obese. (See Chapter 8 for more about obesity and cardiovascular risk factors.)

If you've just learned that you have diabetes, you might feel especially inspired to tackle the challenge of losing weight. After all, improving your health may be of utmost importance now. So make this your motivation and go for it!

Fortunately, most of the meal-planning tools used to create a healthy diabetic diet can also help you to cut back calories. Work with your dietitian to find ways to reduce your caloric intake without starving yourself or skipping a meal. You should also look for ways to squeeze more activity into your daily routine.

Other Tips for Losing Weight

Getting your weight under control is so important to your health when you have diabetes. Below are some tips for how to achieve this critical goal:

- *Think before you eat.* Don't reach mindlessly for your food. Instead, plan and calculate the best foods for your health, trying to always concentrate on boosting your intake of fruits, vegetables, and whole grain foods. At the same time, try to keep fats, sugar, and salt to a minimum.
- *Make sure you eat only when you're hungry.* Do you often eat out of boredom? Stress? Nervousness? Try to get a handle on emotional eating, which can add unwanted calories to your day. If you feel an urge to eat, try taking a brisk ten-minute walk instead. You'll not only dodge the unwanted calories, but you'll burn a few extra ones.
- *Consider keeping a food diary.* A daily record of what and when you eat will help you identify food triggers and high-calorie treats you might be sneaking.
- *Anticipate and plan for challenges.* Headed out to a party? Or dinner at a friend's? Brace yourself by making plans for how you'll stick to your eating plan. Offset an evening of indulgence with smaller meals earlier in the day.
- *Do make room for treats, like dessert.* Deprivation isn't part of a healthy diet, even one that's designed to help you lose weight. So indulge yourself on occasion with a small serving of your favorite cake or pie. Just be careful not to overdo it.

What About Alcohol?

People with diabetes need to take extra precautions if they want to imbibe, but if blood sugar levels are under control, there's no reason why they can't indulge in an occasional drink. But before you do, it's a good idea to talk to your doctor about any possible risks. Often, the doctor's opinion will reflect his own views about drinking alcohol. If your doctor is one who enjoys an occasional drink, he may be inclined to say it's okay for you to have one, too. But if your doctor is a teetotaler, he may recommend you avoid alcohol altogether.

Alcohol can cause low blood sugar in diabetics if it's consumed on an empty stomach. Normally, blood glucose levels drop when your stomach is empty. To avoid a low blood sugar reaction, the liver goes to work, changing stored carbohydrates into glucose, which is then released into your bloodstream. If alcohol enters the body on an empty stomach, the liver won't convert the carbs into glucose. Alcohol reduces the liver's production of glucose, causing blood sugar to decrease. If you have a glass of wine, which contains a lot of sugar, the blood glucose level may actually increase for a while at first, but then will plummet as the liver's production of glucose decreases. You may experience hypoglycemia. But if the wine is taken with a snack or meal, you'll be less likely to develop low blood glucose.

Your odds for low blood sugar are even greater if you drink alcohol after exercising. After a workout, your body is busy replenishing the energy your muscles burned by retrieving glucose from the blood. Taking insulin or diabetes pills with alcohol can also exacerbate your risk for low blood sugar because both treatments work to remove glucose from the blood.

So if you do want to have a drink, enjoy it with food, and keep it to a minimum. Stick with drinks that are lower in alcohol and sugar, such as light beer, a dry wine, or a mixer that contains tonic water, club soda, water, or seltzer. Women should drink no more than one drink at a time, and men should have no more than two. One drink is a twelve-ounce beer or wine cooler, four ounces of wine, or a mixed drink that contains one and a half ounces of liquor.

Besides being hazardous to your health, too much alcohol can impair your judgment and cause you to forget your medications. It can harm the liver and its ability to produce glucose. It also promotes weight gain because it's high in calories.

Avoid alcohol altogether however, if you have nerve damage from your diabetes. Drinking can make the pain even worse. You should also skip the alcohol if you have diabetic eye disease or high blood pressure.

When Routines Are Broken

All the planning in the world can't account for all the changes in your daily schedule that can occur. Below are some possible situations that could interfere with your usual meal plans.

- *A busy workday keeps you at the office later than usual.* Always keep a snack on hand if your job is the kind that can make you late for dinner, or you're likely to get stuck in traffic. Make sure to account for it when you add up the day's carb intake.
- *You went out to dinner with friends and wound up overeating more than your plan allows.* Relax, an occasional splurge happens to everyone, and blood sugar levels can and do fluctuate, no matter how disciplined you are. Rather than fret over a bout of overeating, consider taking a longer walk either before or after the outing to compensate. Or drink an extra glass of water to help the kidneys get rid of the extra sugar in you bloodstream.
- *You're going to eat at a new friend's house and don't know what to expect.* Try to find out beforehand what she's serving, when she'll serve it, and then plan ahead. You might also offer to bring an appetizer or dish, so you can ensure you'll have at least one healthy, low-carb item on the menu.
- *Your children drag you to a fast-food restaurant for lunch, and you're starving.* Steer clear of extra sauces, dressings, or cheese. Avoid fried super-sized packaging, and too much soda. Instead, choose salads with low-cal dressings, kid-sized portions, and lowfat milk or water.

- *You're taking a long-awaited vacation that will probably disrupt your meal plan.* Before you leave, talk things over with your registered dietitian about the food choices you might have and how to adjust your medication if you're crossing time zones. Also, be sure to keep a stash of healthy snacks and bottled water with you, along with your medications and monitoring supplies. It's hard to control when and what you'll eat, so you'll want to be prepared for delays.

The Exercise Component

No healthy lifestyle would be complete without exercise, especially if you have diabetes. Diabetics require physical activity to keep their blood glucose under control and help them lose weight.

But for many people, getting exercise is a challenge. We drive to the office rather than ride our bikes or walk. We take the elevator, instead of the stairs. We mow our laws on riders that require no pushing. And in our free time, we lounge around on couches, glued to the television, rather than engage in activities that get us moving.

All these habits encourage weight gain, which makes you more susceptible to the complications of diabetes. That's why every diabetic needs to exercise. Before getting involved in a fitness program, you need to talk to your physician or exercise physiologist. Some complications of diabetes can inhibit your activity levels and limit your choices. For instance, it's not a good idea to exercise if you already have kidney or nerve damage. Your doctor may also test you for cardiac problems or retinopathy, which can limit your activity. If you're pregnant, you may have to be cautious about overexertion. Again, whatever you choose to do, consult your doctor first.

Why Exercise Matters

Everyone benefits from exercise. Our bodies were designed to move, not to sit before a computer or television for extended hours. For people with diabetes, exercise has the added benefit of making your body cells more sensitive to insulin, thereby helping to remove glucose from your blood. Regular physical activity can also spur weight loss, which is critical for diabetics.

Different kinds of activity affect the body in different ways. Some may actually involve risks, which you should always discuss with your doctor. Here are the three basic kinds:

Cardiovascular

Just as the name implies, cardiovascular, or aerobic, exercise works your heart. You breathe harder, so your lungs also benefit. These exercises can improve blood flow, burn calories, and lower blood pressure, triglycerides, and LDL cholesterol, while raising HDL cholesterol.

Cardiovascular workouts also give you more energy and endurance. Popular cardiovascular exercises include walking, jogging, swimming, tennis, and bicycling.

Strength Training

You may not want the sculpted look of a body builder, but toning your body with weights can do wonders for your health. Weight training strengthens bones and staves off osteoporosis. It also builds muscle, which burns more calories than fat, and keeps your metabolism at a higher rate. In addition, the muscle helps you keep your glucose levels in check. Strength training may be done on weight machines, free weights, or with calisthenics.

Flexibility Exercises

Stretches that improve your range of motion help you adapt to other exercises more quickly and easily. They're a good way to warm up the body and reduce your risk of injuries. You can learn flexibility movements in books, tapes, exercise classes, with a personal trainer, or through yoga.

A Special Note on Walking

You can't beat walking when it comes to ease. It takes no special equipment or training, you don't need a gym, and you can do it literally anywhere. All it requires is a good pair of walking shoes. Best of all, with walking, you're not likely to suffer any injuries.

If it's been years since you picked up a tennis racket or plunged into a swimming pool, you might want to start exercising by walking. Work with your doctor or exercise physiologist to develop an exercise plan. To make sure you don't overdo it, start slowly and gradually progress to a more rigorous walk.

The Effect on Blood Glucose

Done in the right conditions, exercise lowers blood glucose levels to healthier levels. But in some cases, exercise can have a more dramatic impact on blood glucose. That's why you always have to check your blood glucose levels before you exercise.

A safe range is between 100 and 250 mg/dl. If your blood glucose level is below 100 mg/dl, eat a snack that contains at least fifteen grams of carbohydrates, such as an apple. Re-measure your blood glucose fifteen to thirty minutes later, making sure it's at 100 mg/dl or higher before exercising.

If your blood sugar is above 300 mg/dl, don't exercise. A blood sugar above 300 often means you are dehydrated and you need to drink more water. Measure it again and wait until it dips to a safe range. If you have Type 1 diabetes, and your blood sugar is 250 mg/dl, check your urine for ketones. Moderate to high levels of ketones means you should not exercise.

Special Concerns for Insulin Users

For diabetics who take insulin, exercise can affect blood glucose in disparate ways. When you engage in mild or moderate exercise for a short duration, your blood sugar is apt to fall during and after your workout. As you exercise, your body takes up the glucose in your blood to convert it into energy for your cells.

But let's say you exercise for a long period of time or started out on an empty stomach or slightly lower levels of blood glucose. Then you might be at risk for having a bout of hypoglycemia, or low blood sugar. You might feel light-headed or weak. Stop exercising immediately and eat a fast-acting snack that will give your body the sugar it needs. If you want to resume the activity, eat the snack, and wait fifteen minutes.

Sometimes insulin-dependent diabetics may experience high blood glucose levels because they didn't use enough insulin or exercised too long. During bouts of rigorous exercise or in the absence of enough insulin, the liver may start releasing glucose stores, which in turn, will set off the production of ketones. The overproduction of ketones can be dangerous and lead to diabetic ketoacidosis, a potentially life-threatening condition (see Chapter 7).

In general, you should know how fast your insulin works, and then time your workouts according to your meals and injections, or vice versa. If you use short- or rapid-acting insulin for instance, be sure to wait an hour before exercising. Working out before then can cause blood sugar levels to dip too low. As a general rule, avoid physical activity when the insulin is at its peak.

Also, choose your insulin injection site carefully. If you inject it near a muscle that you'll be exerting, the insulin might be absorbed more rapidly and again, blood glucose levels could plummet.

Finally, beware of hypoglycemia in the twenty-four hours after a workout. The possibility of low blood sugar in that time is still higher than normal. So keep glucose tablets or other fast-acting snacks or juices at hand.

Basic Exercise Safety Rules
Here are some rules you should follow in order to stay safe while you exercise.

- *Always do a warm-up and a cool down.* Muscles that have been warmed up are less likely to get injured. So do some stretching before you start exercising.
- *Drink plenty of water before, during, and after exercise.* The fluids will replenish those that are lost during your workout.
- *Pay attention to your breathing.* During weight training or calisthenics, some people forget to breathe. But you need the oxygen to keep you going.
- *Check your feet for cuts, breaks, and swelling.* Diabetics are at risk for poor circulation and neuropathy or nerve damage, which can leave your feet vulnerable to infections you won't necessarily feel. If you're doing an exercise that involves a lot of footwork, you may want to give your feet added protection with cushioned socks. Be sure the shoes you wear to exercise in are also properly fitted.
- *Wear diabetes identifications, if you're away from home.* In the event of hypoglycemia, other people will need that information to help you.
- *Carry glucose tablets, raisins, or fruit juice* for a quick sugar fix in the event of low blood sugar.
- *Don't go alone.* A short trek around the block is one thing, but if you're going on an extended hike in the woods or swimming in a pool, make sure there are other people around who can help in case of a medical emergency.

Get Moving!

For some people, it really is hard to find the time to exercise. Certain days just seem impossibly stacked with appointments and things to do. On those days, look for ways to incorporate exercise into your routine. Here are some ideas:

- Park far away from entrances. Whether it's a supermarket or the doctor's office, pick a spot that will force you to walk.

- Visit colleagues and neighbors in person, instead of using the phone or email.
- Take the stairs, not the elevator.
- Walk through every aisle of the supermarket.
- Do errands on foot whenever you can.
- Rake, mow, and garden.
- Walk inside the bank or restaurant, and avoid the drive-through.

Stay Motivated

Until exercise becomes part of your daily routine, it's easy to skip a workout and do something else. After all, you're busy. On some days, finding time to exercise might seem like an impossible challenge.

But now that you know you have diabetes, you should make an extra effort to get moving. Here are some tips to help you sustain your interest level:

- *Choose activities you enjoy.* Don't take on tennis, for example, if you hate competitive sports. Don't try swimming if the water bothers your skin. Instead, select activities that you will enjoy doing, so you'll improve the chances that you'll stick with them.
- *Write it on your calendar.* Make a date with yourself to exercise. If you write it down like you would any other appointment, you'll be more apt to stick with it and not allow other things to interfere.
- *Consider enlisting a workout buddy.* If you prefer the companionship of your spouse or a friend, ask that person to join you on your exercise. Having someone with you will help you pass the time and make your exercise more enjoyable.
- *Set specific goals.* Make sure you set both short- and long-term goals. Initial short-term goals might be walking ten minutes a day three times a week for the next two weeks or doing fifteen

minutes of weight training twice a week. A long-term goal might be trying to lose eight pounds in two months.

- *Reward yourself for your progress.* Seeing the progress you've made will help you stay motivated, but toss in a tangible reward as a gift to yourself. Buy a new pair of walking shoes, go see a show, or treat yourself to a massage. You've earned it!
- *Spice things up with variety.* Doing the same workout day after day will eventually get boring. So jazz things up with some variations. Take a different route on your walk. Add some new moves to your yoga routine. Experiment with classes.

Make It a Habit

Exercising on weekends only or once in a while isn't enough to make a difference when it comes to losing weight or lowering your blood glucose levels. What diabetics—and really everyone for that matter—need to do is make physical activity a daily part of their lives. Exercise is an insulin sensitizer and makes the sugar go into the muscle cells. No medication can do what exercise does for increasing glucose uptake in the muscle cells. Even better, the effects of exercise often last more than twelve hours.

But making exercise a regular habit isn't easy for everyone. Some people dislike exercise and dread the thought of working out. Others manage to do it, but can't stick with a routine. And we all certainly have periods in our lives when we really are too busy to squeeze in a good workout.

That's okay. The key is to keep doing it whenever you can, as often as you can, even if it means doing it in short five- or ten-minute spurts for a time. Try to reinforce your new habit by reading about the health benefits of exercise, surrounding yourself with other people who enjoy exercising, and keeping a journal of how the added activity makes you feel.

Then, just do it! It can take up to six months to build a new habit, but the rewards are well worth it. Besides losing weight and getting better control of your glucose levels, you'll sleep better, have more energy, and reduce your stress. All these factors will contribute to a better quality of life.

CHAPTER FIVE

All About Insulin

Getting a handle on blood sugar by eating a healthy diet and getting regular exercise is great—if you can do it. But if you have Type 1 diabetes or you no longer produce enough insulin, you will become dependent on insulin.

Injecting yourself with a shot several times a day may seem daunting to you at first, possibly even scary. But like the oxygen you breathe and the water you drink, insulin is essential to your survival. Developing a better understanding of what it is and why you need it will help you appreciate its importance. And becoming familiar with the different types of insulin and the various options for administration will help you find the best way to get insulin inside your bloodstream.

What Is Insulin?

Inside the pancreas of a healthy person, in the islets of Langerhans, beta cells busily churn out the hormone insulin throughout the day; it falls and rises as your needs change. Whenever blood glucose levels rise, such as after a meal, the hormone goes to work. Like a key, insulin acts on insulin receptors on the surface of cells and sends messages to glucose transport proteins, which allow glucose to enter the cells and be converted into energy for our bodies. The process helps eliminate glucose from the blood.

Insulin also plays a role in the storage of extra glucose by the liver. When insulin levels are high, the liver accepts and stores extra glucose in the form of glycogen, thereby removing it from the bloodstream. When insulin levels are low, the liver releases glycogen into the blood as sugar for extra energy. The constant ebb and flow of glycogen from the liver also helps keep blood sugar at normal levels.

In people who have Type 1 diabetes, the pancreas no longer makes insulin. People who have Type 2 diabetes sometimes don't produce enough insulin. Without insulin, the glucose can't get inside the insulin sensitive cells and instead is left to linger in the bloodstream. There, it travels through the body, causing glucose toxicity. Having high blood glucose levels is the cause of diabetes.

Only by getting insulin into the bloodstream are you able to move the glucose out of the blood. But insulin cannot be taken orally because the digestive process would destroy it. Instead, insulin must be injected into the body by syringe, pen, or a pump.

History of Insulin

It took years for scientists to discover and perfect the use of insulin for the treatment of diabetes. Before its discovery in 1922, diabetics were starved and given large amounts of fluid in futile efforts to control their diabetes. Some were treated with opium, special diets, or bloodletting. Of course, these treatments failed, and most diabetics died within years after they were diagnosed.

Then in 1922, Frederick Banting, a Canadian surgeon, and Charles Best, a medical student, discovered insulin using experiments on a dog. Months later, they treated their first human patient, a fourteen-year-old boy named Leonard Thompson. Once emaciated and wasted, Thompson soon began to gain weight and went on to live another fifteen years.

But it was years before the production of insulin was perfected. At first, insulin was available only from pigs and cows. These fast-acting insulins from animals were used up quickly and were often unreliable in strength and purity. They also produced allergic reactions and caused irritations at the injection site.

Eventually, in the 1980s, scientists were able to produce human insulin in laboratories, using the human insulin gene and bacteria from the pancreas. The gene is placed inside the bacteria, where it instructs the bacteria to manufacture insulin. Today, this synthetic form of human insulin is the most widely used form. Animal insulin, specifically that from pigs, is used primarily in patients who were diagnosed years ago and whose blood glucose is now well-controlled by porculine insulin. Bovine insulin from cows is no longer available.

The Different Kinds of Insulin

Diabetics have more than twenty types of insulin to choose from, in four basic forms. Each one has a different time of onset, peak, and duration of action. Onset time is the time it takes for the insulin to get into the blood and start lowering blood glucose. Peak time refers to the point at which the insulin is at its maximal strength. Duration is the length of time in which the insulin continues to function. Choosing the right one for you will depend on your lifestyle, blood sugar levels, and injection site, as well as your physician's preference.

- *Rapid-acting insulin* has an onset time of fifteen minutes, with peak action at thirty to ninety minutes. The effect typically last three to five hours. Some examples include Humalog (lispro) and Novolog (aspart). The fast action means patients can easily time their insulin to their meals. These insulins are also called insulin analogs.
- *Short-acting insulin,* also called regular insulin, goes into action in thirty to sixty minutes, peaks between fifty and one hundred

and twenty minutes and can last from five to eight hours. Regular insulin was the first kind available. Examples include Humulin R and Novolin R.

- *Intermediate-acting insulin* has an onset time of one to three hours, peaks at eight hours, and can last as long as twenty hours. Among the brands of intermediate-acting insulin are Humulin N and Novolin N.

- *Long-acting insulin* takes more time to work, as much as eight hours. Some brands peak between eight and twelve hours, but others may have no peak time. The duration time is anywhere from twenty-four to thirty-six hours. An example of a long-acting insulin is Ultralente, which has a relatively flat-acting duration, but in larger doses—above twenty-five units—may have a slight peak between eight to twelve hours.

- *New long-acting insulin analogs* provide a more constant release of insulin into the fatty tissue. The first insulin of this kind is called glargine (Lantus) U-100 insulin, which behaves much like the way an insulin pump does when it administers basal insulin, the steady, constant flow of insulin that is present in healthypeople. It has a pH of 4.0 and therefore, must not be mixed with other insulin preparations. Glargine is a true twenty-four-hour insulin and can be given once a day. It may be given at bedtime or in the morning when you are taking your rapid-acting insulin. Some diabetics call the combination of glargine as a basal insulin and lispro or aspart as rapid-acting insulin before each meal the "convenience pump." This protocol can be used in both Type 1 and other diabetics when indicated. Similar to an insulin pump, it allows for more predictability in the insulin action and less demand to eat at certain times of the day.

In general, the slower-acting insulins require fewer doses a day. Sometimes one at breakfast and one at bedtime is all you need. The rapid-acting insulin can help you make on-the-spot adjustments to blood glucose levels if, for instance, you decide to eat an extra helping of pasta. You may also be at lower risk for hypoglycemia because the insulin doesn't stay in your body as long.

Sometimes, your doctor will recommend that you use a mixture of intermediate- and short-acting insulins. You can buy a mixture that has a 50/50 mixture or one with 70 percent intermediate-acting insulin and 30 percent regular insulin. Your doctor may also use a mix of Ultralente U, a long-acting insulin, and Semilente, a regular insulin. Mixed in a 70/30 percent ratio, the two produce Lente L insulin, which is similar to NPH, an intermediate-acting insulin. These brands have been largely replaced by the newer analog insulins and NPH, but are still used in patients who are allergic to NPH.

You may have the option of mixing the insulins yourself. But be sure to consult your doctor before attempting to mix different types of insulin.

Choosing the Right Regimen

Besides figuring out which insulin to take, you also need to determine how often to take it. Some people with diabetes may require a single dose of an intermediate-acting insulin every day. Others will require a split dose, or two injections of intermediate-acting insulin a day, which are usually administered before breakfast and dinner. Or you may have to take a split mixed dose that combines a short-acting and intermediate-acting insulin. For some people, especially Type 1 diabetics, intensive insulin therapy is needed to tightly regulate blood sugar and keep it near the normal range.

What Is Intensive Insulin Therapy?

With intensive insulin therapy, your goal is to mimic the way insulin is naturally secreted by the pancreas. In a healthy person, the pancreas secretes insulin throughout the day, releasing higher levels only if there's more glucose in the blood. So it isn't just a matter of taking more insulin, but rather adjusting it to accommodate everyday changes in your diet, activity level, and blood glucose levels. Intensive insulin therapy is often recommended for Type 1 diabetics and women with gestational diabetes who need to have tight control of blood sugars.

But intensive insulin therapy isn't without risks. People who tightly regulate blood glucose are at risk for hypoglycemia because they're striving to keep their blood glucose levels in the near normal range. They're also more likely to gain weight. With more insulin in the blood, you'll be moving more glucose into body cells. And if that glucose isn't converted into energy, it will be stored as fat.

Getting Insulin into the Body

Currently, the only way to get insulin into your bloodstream is by injection. Taking it orally is not an option because the digestive process will render it ineffective. But you do have some options in terms of how to inject it.

Syringe

Not long ago, the only way you could inject insulin was to use a syringe. Though the syringe is still the most common method of injection, it is now considerably easier to use, with smooth silicon-coated needles that make the injections less painful and plastic materials that make for easy disposal.

The syringe basically consists of a needle, barrel, and plunger. It works by drawing insulin out of a bottle, and then injecting the insulin into fatty tissue under your skin (more on injection sites later). Today's modern needles are covered with a special coating that makes it less painful to insert into the skin.

When choosing a syringe, make sure the syringe size matches the strength of the insulin. Most diabetics use a strength of U-100, meaning the insulin contains 100 units of insulin in every cubic centimeter of fluid. It's also important that the syringe is large enough to hold a single dose of insulin. Syringes now come in 0.3cc, 0.5cc and 1.0cc. This allows for more accurate measurements in diabetics requiring smaller amounts of insulin.

In addition, you should make sure that the dosage lines on your syringe closely correspond with the dose you need to measure. The lines on some syringes indicate one unit, while others have lines that equal two units. The lines should also be easy to read.

Some patients reuse their syringes in the interest of saving money or producing less medical waste. The choice to do so is entirely up to you. If you wish to reuse your syringe, you should recap it and avoid letting it touch anything except your clean skin. Store the syringe at room temperature. Do not wipe the needle with alcohol since that can remove the coating that makes the needle smooth. Insulin already contains some antibacterial substances that protects against bacterial growth.

But you should not reuse syringes if the needle is bent or dull. A good rule would be to use a new needle and syringe when possible. You should also avoid reusing a syringe if you have poor hygiene, are ill, have open wounds, or have a low resistance to infection. It is also not a good idea to reuse a syringe with a different kind of insulin than the one you used before. Trace amounts of the first insulin always remain on the needle. Most important, you should never, ever use another patient's syringe or allow someone to use yours.

When you do discard a syringe, do it carefully. A used syringe is considered medical waste. Putting your used syringes with needles into a plastic container and placing a cap on the container before throwing it into your regular trash is recommended and meets regulatory guidelines for most states. It should never be tossed directly into a trash can since it contains traces of human blood.

Other Injection Devices

Syringes aren't the only way to inject insulin. You might talk to your doctor about some of these other alternatives:

- *Automatic injectors.* If you have trouble actually inserting the needle into your skin, you might consider an injector. With an automatic injector, the touch of a button automatically shoots the needle into your skin. Some injectors even dispense the insulin at that point. With others, you still need to use the syringe.
- *Jet injectors.* These contraptions spare you the use of needles altogether. The jet injector works by quickly injecting a dosage of insulin into the skin. The problem with this device is it's costly and involves more maintenance for cleaning. A good cleaning requires taking apart the injector and boiling it for sterilization or using germicidal cleaners, which are potentially irritating. There's also a problem with bruising in children, thin people, and the elderly. Most patients experience pain from the use of a jet injector.
- *Pen injectors.* These devices resemble pens, but instead of a writing tip, the pen injector has a needle. Inside the pen, there's a cartridge of insulin that delivers the dosage according to the settings on the injector. Pen injectors have two key advantages: They're highly portable, and once the cartridge is empty, they're easily disposed of.
- *Infusers.* You can reduce the number of times you poke yourself with a needle using an infuser. Infusers are tiny catheters inserted under the skin that stay in place with tape for up to three days. Whenever you need insulin, you inject the needle into the infuser. Although less painful, the infuser can raise the risk for local infection.

Injection Sites

Whether it's a syringe or an injection pen, you need to choose where to inject the insulin into your body. The site must be an area that contains enough fat since the needle is inserted directly into the fat above the muscle.

Most diabetics inject into the abdomen, making sure to avoid the area around the navel. In the abdomen, the insulin is absorbed most quickly and at the most consistent speed. You may also choose to inject into the upper and outer thighs, backs of the upper arms, the thighs, or the buttocks. The arms absorb the insulin more slowly than the abdomen, and the hips or buttocks are even slower.

Once you decide where to inject, follow these basic guidelines:

- *Space your injections apart from one another.* Make sure each one is at least a finger width away from your last shot.
- *Avoid injecting into muscles.*
- *Try administering all your shots in one region of the body.* Different sites absorb insulin at different rates. Sticking with one region, such as the abdomen, helps you maintain better control of your insulin.
- *Don't inject too close to a mole or scar tissue.*
- *If you do choose the abdomen,* avoid injecting anywhere in a two-inch radius around the navel, where the tougher tissue can cause erratic insulin absorption.
- *If you decide to inject into your thighs,* steer clear of the knees, where there is less fat. Also, avoid the inner thighs, where rubbing can cause pain and friction.
- *Work with your doctor or diabetes educator* on developing a rotation plan that matches your own lifestyle. By rotating the sites of your injections, you can adjust your insulin levels to accommodate your lifestyle. For instance, if you go to bed early, you might want your insulin to sustain you through the long night. You can achieve a slower absorption rate by injecting into the thighs.
- *Be careful about injections before you exercise.* Strenuous exercise on the muscles near the injection site can speed up the absorption rate of insulin. The fast absorption combined with exercise can put you at risk for hypoglycemia.

Problems at the Injection Site

When you first begin to inject insulin, you may notice some redness or swelling at the injection site. Sometimes, there are impurities in the insulin or traces of alcohol still on the site from cleaning it. Be sure to let the area air dry before making the injection.

These problems usually disappear in two to three weeks, but can often cause pain in the meantime. To minimize the pain, be sure you're relaxed when administering the shot. Make sure the insulin is at room temperature and that there are no air bubbles in the syringe. Air bubbles do not cause air embolisms, but can lead to inaccuracy in the amount of insulin you get. Insert the needle quickly, and keep it in one direction.

Sometimes, you may notice dents in the skin at the injection site. This is called lipoatrophy and results from the disappearance of fatty tissue under the skin. Although it's unclear why it occurs, your body is having an immune reaction and responding to the insulin as a foreign substance. Lipoatrophy doesn't usually occur with human insulin, so make sure you're using highly purified human insulin.

Another problem that may occur is hypertrophy, the overgrowth of fat cells. The skin winds up looking lumpy. The solution is not to change insulin, but to switch to a different injection site. Sometimes, you can develop lipohypertrophy, a buildup of fat deposits caused by using the same sites over and over again.

Your best bet for avoiding these problems is to rotate the site of your injections. The abnormal cell growth can inhibit the absorption of insulin and cause problems with your blood glucose control. Speak to your doctor about developing a good site rotation plan.

How Many Shots a Day?

The number of injections you administer daily will depend on your health, the type of insulin you're using, and how well-controlled your blood glucose is. Type 1 diabetics are dependent on insulin for survival and will often need several shots a day. Some Type 2 diabetics may not need insulin at all because they can achieve blood glucose control simply through diet and exercise. But others may need one or two shots of insulin to help them get a better handle on blood glucose. The same is true of women who have gestational diabetes.

In patients who need tighter control, several shots are usually needed every day. These patients may require a long-acting shot of insulin for baseline or basal coverage, which provides a steady stream of insulin throughout the day and night. Then at meals, they'll need to take a shot of rapid-acting insulin to cover the surge in blood glucose following the intake of food.

Another way to ensure 24/7 insulin coverage is by mixing rapid- and short-acting insulin with intermediate-acting insulins and injecting them in two shots, before breakfast and dinner. The rapid- and short-acting insulins kick in to cover breakfast, then subside just as the intermediate-acting insulin goes into action. Shortly before dinner, a second dose of the mix is given, and a similar pattern occurs at dinner time. The intermediate-acting insulin then lingers on to cover your insulin needs overnight.

Some patients may require three shots a day, such as those who are prone to low blood glucose in the early morning. Taking a mix of short- and intermediate-acting insulin at breakfast will provide coverage through most of the day. Follow it up with a shot of short-acting insulin at dinner to cover needs at the evening meal. A third shot of intermediate-acting insulin before bed will help avoid low blood glucose levels in the middle of the night between 2 and 4 am. Bedtime injections of intermediate or long-acting insulin can help reduce the high blood glucose levels that may occur overnight. The increased production of growth hormones in those hours can raise blood glucose between 4 and 6 am, an occurrence called the dawn phenomenon.

The mix and dose schedule will vary, depending on your needs. But keep in mind that more frequent injections mean greater opportunities for control. No matter what the schedule, it's critical to continue doing frequent blood glucose checks. Your readings can tell you whether to have an injection before a meal (if blood glucose is too high) or after a meal (if blood glucose is too low).

Insulin Pumps

Since their advent in the 1960s, pumps have evolved from large, clunky devices into small portable gadgets that are easily hooked onto the waistband and resemble a pager. Not surprisingly, they have become more popular in recent years.

Pumps imitate the action of insulin in healthy people by delivering a steady dose of insulin all through the day and a larger jolt of insulin whenever blood glucose levels rise. The technical name is continuous subcutaneous insulin infusion or CSII. A small needle is inserted in the skin beneath fatty tissue and taped into place. The needle is attached to a catheter that connects to the pump, where the insulin is stored.

The insulin is delivered by slow infusion at a rate determined by your doctor that depends on your metabolism. This slow, steady infusion provides the basal coverage, and flows continuously day and night. Then, before you eat, you can push a button that delivers extra insulin from the pump, which is called the bolus. The bolus can be easily adjusted to accommodate the amount of carbohydrates you plan to eat. Consider the bolus an insulin injection without the needle.

The pump offers many advantages. It provides greater flexibility in terms of eating since you're adjusting the insulin dosage to match the meal. For many patients, it's also easy to use. Rather than filling a syringe, you simply push a button. You can even remove the pump for an hour or two if you're going to engage in physical activities that suppress blood glucose levels. But keep in mind that you may need an injection during that time if the exercise isn't rigorous enough.

Pumps are also extremely precise, delivering exact amounts of insulin down to the tenth of a unit for patients who need maximum control over blood glucose. And whenever you're out of insulin, the battery is low, or the line is clogged, your pump will sound an alarm to alert you.

But the pump does have disadvantages. For one, it's expensive. A pump can cost as much as $7,500, with monthly maintenance expenses as high as $300 for insulin, infusion sets, and blood testing supplies. You should check whether your insurance company will cover these costs if you're interested in purchasing a pump.

Also, convenient as it is, the pump needs maintenance. You need to remove the catheter every two or three days to change the infusion site. You also have to refill the reservoir that holds the insulin every few days. These may seem minor however, compared to the routine injections of insulin every day.

As remarkable as it is, the pump still cannot sense your body's blood glucose levels and does not erase the need for you to monitor. You'll still need to take frequent blood glucose checks to make sure your pump is supplying the right amount of insulin.

Should I Use a Pump?

Despite its assets, not everyone needs to use a pump or even wants a pump. If your blood glucose levels are being well managed by injections, it might not be worth the time and money to learn how to use a pump.

But some people can benefit greatly from a pump, especially if they're looking to achieve tight control of their blood glucose. Women who are pregnant or trying to become pregnant for instance, might consider a pump since high blood glucose can endanger their health as well as the well-being of their unborn baby. Babies born to mothers with diabetes are at risk for birth defects and illness, though the risk is the same as that for non-diabetic moms if blood glucose is well-controlled before and during pregnancy.

You might also consider a pump if you've had difficulties regulating blood sugar and are prone to episodes of hypoglycemia or hyperglycemia.

If your lifestyle is one that varies a great deal from day to day, a pump can make it more convenient to adjust your insulin to your changing needs.

If you do decide to try a pump, talk it over with your doctor and diabetes educator. You need to have a clear understanding of how your diet and activities can impact blood glucose and know how insulin can help control blood glucose. You also have to feel comfortable with operating a pump. The pump works only as well as the person who controls it.

Your Insulin Supply

Insulins come in different strengths and are purchased from a pharmacy. Most people use U-100 insulin, meaning there are 100 units of insulin per milliliter of fluid. You should get your insulin from the same pharmacy where you get all your medications. You should also get all your insulin from one pharmacy, which ensures you'll get the same type and concentration each time.

Once, you have the insulin, read the instruction label for information on storage and use. In general, insulin is stored in the refrigerator until you need it. Write down the date you opened it. You can store the opened bottle at room temperature for up to a month. Beyond that time, insulin can become less potent and should be discarded. Opened bottles kept in the refrigerator can be kept for up to three months. Also keep an eye on the expiration date, and throw away any bottle that is expired.

Don't store insulin in places with extreme temperatures. Cold insulin can be painful upon injection. If insulin is kept in temperatures below 36 degrees, it's also apt to clump. Likewise, avoid storing insulin in hot temperatures or placing it in direct sunlight. Insulin spoils if it's kept in temperatures above 86 degrees.

Before using any insulin, check it over carefully. If it contains clumps or particles, or has a change in color, don't use it. Some insulins, like NPH and Lente, are cloudy in appearance, and need to be rolled up to twenty times to get a good mix. Shaking it however, can cause the insulin to clump and destroy its effectiveness. Other kinds are clear. Be familiar with how your insulin should look. The insulin may very well be contaminated or have lost its potency. That's why you should always keep an extra bottle on hand.

The Future of Insulin

Someday, you may be able to absorb your insulin from a patch, inhale it into your lungs by way of an aerosol, or ingest it in the form of pills. Scientists are researching alternative methods for delivering insulin into the bloodstream that may someday render the needle and syringe method obsolete. Researchers are also looking at developing an artificial pancreas that could be implanted in the abdominal cavity and an oral spray that would deliver insulin through the mucous membranes of the cheeks, tongue, and throat. But extensive testing still needs to go on before these products make it onto the marketplace.

Getting a Handle on Insulin

Working closely with your doctor, you'll be able to determine the type or types of insulin you'll need, the amount you need to take, a schedule for taking it, and how you'll administer the insulin. Whether you're practicing standard therapy and injecting insulin once or twice a day or intensive therapy and injecting insulin three or more times a day, you will need some time and practice to iron out any kinks. Don't hesitate to discuss any concerns or problems with your doctor or diabetes educator. Chances are, they'll be able to guide you as you perfect your insulin plan.

CHAPTER SIX 🌿

Oral Medications for Diabetes

For some people with insulin resistance and Type 2 diabetes, changing your diet and losing fifteen pounds is enough to bring blood glucose levels under control. For others, it might be adopting a new exercise regimen and sticking with it regularly. But in some people with Type 2 diabetes, these lifestyle changes still don't make a dent, and their physician may prescribe an oral medication to lower blood glucose.

Diabetics can choose from six categories of medications, all of which must be prescribed by your doctor. Different drugs work in different ways. Some stimulate the pancreas to produce more insulin. Others help your body become less resistant to the effects of insulin. Others slow your body's absorption of carbohydrates.

In this chapter, we'll take a look at the different kinds of medications for diabetes. But taking medication doesn't mean you can go back to an unhealthy diet or give up your exercise routine. Even with medications, you must still stick to a healthy diet and get some regular exercise. You may even need to take insulin if your doctor decides it's necessary. Only by combining all the components of your treatment plan will you be able to get control of your blood glucose.

Why You Might Need Drugs

You're already eating a healthy diet and exercising regularly. You might have even lost a few pounds. But still your blood glucose levels refuse to drop. That's when your physician might decide you need an oral medication.

Oral medications are usually the first line of attack if you have Type 2 diabetes, and lifestyle changes alone don't work to reduce blood glucose. Pills are considerably easier to take than insulin. They're also less likely to cause hypoglycemia than insulin is. And if you're overweight or obese, you may require large doses of insulin that your doctor might prefer to avoid.

Certain measures of blood glucose may qualify you for medications. If your blood glucose is 140 mg/dl before breakfast, or your bedtime blood glucose is above 160 mg/dl, you may be a candidate for medications. Drugs may also be considered if your HbA1C reading is over 6.5 percent. HbA1C above 6.5 percent is associated with microvascular complications, especially those involving the small blood vessels of the eye. Starting medications at lower blood glucose levels may help slow the progression of the disease and help you better control diabetes before complications develop.

Sulfonylureas

The use of sulfonylureas for diabetes was discovered by accident during World War II when soldiers were given medications containing sulfur as antibiotics. The doctors noticed that the medications lowered blood glucose in the soldiers.

In 1955, pharmaceutical companies began marketing sulfonylureas for the treatment of diabetes in the U.S. And until 1994, they were the only drugs available for the treatment of diabetes in this country. Sulfonylureas work by stimulating the beta cells in the pancreas to produce and release more insulin. In order for sulfonylureas to work, your pancreas must still be making insulin. Today, sulfonylureas are divided up into first- and second-generation versions. The second generation versions are prescribed more frequently these days because they have fewer side effects and interactions with other drugs.

The following is a list of sulfonylureas, with the brand name beside it:

- *Acetohexamide (Dymelor)* is a first-generation sulfonylurea that begins to work an hour after ingestion and lasts up to twelve hours.
- *Chlorpropamide (Diabinese, Glucamide)* has the longest duration of the sulfonylureas and so is less commonly prescribed. The long-lasting effect of this first-generation drug puts the user at greater risk for hypoglycemia than other sulfonylureas.
- *Glimepiride (Amaryl)* is a second-generation sulfonylurea that lasts as long as twenty-four hours. Glimepiride is not available in generic form.
- *Glipizide and Glipizide ER (Glucotrol, Glucotrol XL)* are also second-generation drugs and produce a faster reduction of blood sugar than some of the others. Glipizide ER does not come in a generic form.
- *Glyburide (Diabeta, Glynase, Micronase)* is more potent than glipizide, so patients usually require fewer doses.
- *Tolazamide (Tolinase)* is a second-generation sulfonylurea that doesn't go into effect until up to four hours after you take it. But it also lasts as long as twenty hours.
- *Tolbutamide (Orinase)* is the only short-acting sulfonylurea and is part of the first generation of these medications. It begins to work in an hour and lasts as long as ten hours. The primary advantage of this sulfonylurea is a reduced risk for hypoglycemia.

These drugs are usually taken once or twice a day before meals. But they do produce side effects, such as constipation, diarrhea, cramping, skin rash and itching, increased sensitivity to sunlight, nausea and vomiting, weight gain, and headache.

In some patients, sulfonylureas can cause hypoglycemia, or low blood sugar. You should be familiar with the symptoms of hypoglycemia if you take these medications. You should also always carry a fast-acting carbohydrate food with you at all times if you take a sulfonylurea.

In addition, you should avoid alcohol, which can cause low blood sugar. People who have an allergy to sulfa medications are advised to avoid sulfonylureas altogether.

Biguanides

In 1994, metformin (Glucophage and Glucophage XR) was introduced in the U.S. as another way to treat diabetes by medication. Metformin is the only drug in this class that's available in this country. As a biguanide, metformin acts on the liver by limiting the amount of glucose it releases, thereby lowering your need for insulin. In addition, it decreases the amount of sugar that gets absorbed into your intestines.

Depending on the kind you are prescribed, metformin is taken one to three times a day. Metformin is commonly prescribed to overweight patients because the drug is less likely to cause weight gain than some of the other diabetes medications. It also helps lower blood lipids such as cholesterol and triglycerides. But biguanides can cause other side effects such as an unpleasant metallic taste, loss of appetite, nausea or vomiting, abdominal discomfort, gas or diarrhea, and skin rash. Starting slowly by taking it once per day may reduce the side effects and diarrhea. Most patients can tolerate 500 to 2500 mg per day. The extended release form, Glucophage XR, also reduces the side effects and allows once-a-day administration. The Glucophage XR is in a capsule that does not dissolve, but is rather released through a laser hole in the pill.

If you do use metformin, avoid alcohol. The combination can produce lactic acidosis, a buildup of lactic acid in the blood that can be fatal. The drug also cannot be combined with cimetidine (Tagamet) because cimetidine can interfere with your body's ability to eliminate metformin. A buildup of metformin can cause lactic acidosis.

Alpha-Glucosidase Inhibitors

In 1996, two drugs in this category were approved for use in the U.S.; miglitol (Glyset) and acarbose (Precose). Both medications are taken right before a meal and work by slowing the digestion and absorption of carbohydrates through the small intestine. The effect is a less exaggerated spike in blood glucose after meals, known as postprandial elevations. The drugs also help lower the HbA1C.

Although they're generally safe and effective, they can produce side effects such as abdominal bloating, gas, or diarrhea. The best way to lessen these side effects is to start on a low dose and to gradually increase it. Patients who already have digestive disorders such as Crohn's disease or irritable bowel syndrome should avoid these medications.

Taking miglitol or acarbose with another diabetes medication does also raises your risk for hypoglycemia. If you do have a bout of hypoglycemia, do not treat it with fruit juice or table sugar. These medications inhibit the digestion of these sugars.

Meglitinides (Non-Sulfonylureas)

Another option for diabetics who experience postprandial elevation are the meglitinides. Repaglinide (Prandin) is currently the only drug in this category. Like the sulfonylureas, repaglinide helps lower blood glucose by stimulating the beta cells to release more insulin.

But unlike the sulfonylureas, repaglinide works only in response to a meal. The action is fast, and the effects of the drug are short-lived. Repaglinide is usually taken with the meals to lessen the surge in blood glucose. Like the sulfonylureas, repaglinide does raise the risk for hypoglycemia. You should also avoid taking it with alcohol.

Thiazolidinediones (Glitazones)

People who have developed a resistance to insulin can no longer rely on the hormone to help remove blood glucose. Thiazolidinediones work by making your body tissues more sensitive to insulin. Their effects are primarily on the muscle and fat cells. They may also increase the production of insulin from the pancreas in response to prolonged hyperglycemia. Drugs in this category are rosiglitazone (Avandia) and pioglitazone (Actos). A third drug, troglitazone (Rezulin) was removed from the market in 2000 after several cases of liver failure were linked to its use.

Thiazolidinediones or TZDs, which are taken once or twice a day, have the added benefit of lowering triglycerides and increasing HDL cholesterol, but do also have side effects. These may include swelling, weight gain, and fatigue. Although some patients may be concerned about damage to the liver, to date, no cases of liver failure have been reported that are due to the direct effect of rosiglitazone or pioglitizone. But you may have to undergo blood tests to check the health of your liver before you can be given one of these medications. TZDs are contraindicated in the presence of congestive heart failure and should be given with caution to patients with ischemic heart disease who have angina or shortness of breath while walking.

D-phenylalanine

In 2000, the FDA approved the first drug in this new classification, called nateglinide (Starlix). Nateglinide works by stimulating the rapid production of insulin that is needed right after a meal. The drug is taken about a minute before the meal begins and helps level off postprandial sugar spikes.

One benefit of nateglinide is that it does not linger in the body after the blood glucose is reduced. Its short action span means it lowers the patient's risk for hypoglycemia, which occurred in just 2.4 percent of patients during trials of the drug. In some patients, the drug produced cold-like symptoms.

Combining Medications

Sometimes, one drug is not enough to effectively lower your blood glucose, and your doctor may recommend that you combine two medications. The most common drug used in combination with another are the sulfonylureas. For instance, a sulfonylurea and metformin combination might be prescribed to lower fasting blood sugar and glycated hemoglobin, while also promoting weight loss. Combining a sulfonylurea with a TZD can help boost the effectiveness of the sulfonylurea as it stimulates the production of insulin. In 2000, the FDA approved the marketing of Glucovance, the first combination pill that brings together glyburide, a sulfonylurea, and metformin. Rosiglitizone combined with metformin is available as Avandamet. The combination decreases the release of glucose by the liver, increases the uptake of glucose by fat and muscle, and increases insulin release from the pancreas.

Some patients who use insulin may also have to take medications. Most pills act by improving the body's use of insulin. One likely combination is taking a TZD with insulin. For people with well-controlled blood glucose, the TZD can lower the amount of insulin you need. If your blood glucose is not well-controlled, the TZD can enhance your sensitivity to the insulin. The incidence of leg swelling, called edema, rises when combining insulin with TZDs.

Who Doesn't Benefit

Not everyone will respond positively to an oral medication for diabetes. People who have Type 1 diabetes, for instance, are never prescribed diabetes medications as their primary treatment. If a Type 1 diabetic develops insulin resistance, requires more than forty units of insulin per day, and is overweight, insulin sensitizers will occasionally be added to insulin therapy.

When Certain Meds Are Not Prescribed

Other patients cannot use certain medications because of preexisting conditions or surgery. Some contraindications that require special attention include:

- Metformin is not prescribed in patients with moderate to severe renal insufficiency. It is also not used in acutely ill patients and should be stopped if a diabetic is admitted to a hospital for critical care until the patient is adequately hydrated.
- Metformin is also not used when CAT scans and other imaging procedures are being done because the excretion of the contrast dyes and metformin occurs along the same pathway in the kidney. Using metformin with these dyes may lead to lactic acidosis, and, if not corrected, may cause death in patients with renal insufficiency.
- Although not approved by the FDA for use in pregnancy, metformin has been used in women with polycystic ovarian disease and does appears to be safe in the event they become pregnant.
- Sulfonylureas are generally not used in patients with moderate to severe renal disease and should be replaced with insulin if other oral agents do not work.
- Glyburide is the only sulfonylurea which has published data to support its use for gestational diabetes. It is the only sulfonylurea that does not cross the placenta and does not affect the fetus. Occasionally a pharmacist may substitute one sulfonylurea for another without knowing a patient is pregnant. Pregnant patients should be aware of this possibility. Generally, insulin is the primary treatment for gestational diabetes.
- TZDs are not prescribed if a patient has liver disease and congestive heart failure. But they can be used in patients with renal failure.

When the Drug Doesn't Work

By monitoring your blood glucose carefully, you'll be able to determine whether your medication is working. A clear sign is hyperglycemia, or excess blood glucose. Hyperglycemia shows that the medication is not doing what it's supposed to do, which is to lower blood glucose.

In some patients, the drug may never work at all. Your doctor may need to give you a different prescription or increase the dosage. In other patients, the pills may work well for a while, but then lose their effectiveness. Approximately 5-10 percent of all people who have initial success with a sulfonylurea stop responding within several years. Eventually, another 50 percent will stop responding. When this happens, you might need a different drug, a combination of medications, or insulin. You will need to work with your doctor to determine the next best course of treatment.

Safety Concerns

All medications can cause side effects and harmful interactions when combined with other medicines. Diabetes drugs are no exception. All sulfonylureas, for instance, can raise your risk for hypoglycemia, a potentially life-threatening situation. Oral diabetes medications are also not prescribed to pregnant women. People who develop major infections or are about to undergo surgery usually have to replace their oral medications with insulin for a time.

The only way to prevent a bad reaction or interaction is to tell your doctor and/or pharmacist about other medications you are taking or may take, including vitamins, over-the-counter products, or herbal remedies. Even a seemingly harmless over-the-counter drug can become harmful if it's combined with another medication.

You should follow your doctor's instructions carefully. Be sure you know exactly how much you need to take and when to take it. Be clear about any precautions or special instructions. Ask your doctor about circumstances in which he should be notified.

A PERSONAL STORY

Elaine

Finding the right medication to treat diabetes can sometimes be a challenge. That's what Elaine, a sixty-two-year-old retired nurse found out even after having initial success with a sulfonylurea.

At the time she was diagnosed in 1991, her blood sugars hovered around 200 mg/dl. Her doctor at the time—whom she describes as "very laid back"— didn't want to prescribe any medications and told her to try to rein in her blood glucose with diet and exercise. But diet and exercise didn't work, and Elaine went to another doctor. The second doctor prescribed Diabeta (glyburide), a sulfonylurea that stimulates the beta cells in the pancreas to produce more insulin.

For ten years, the Diabeta worked wonderfully, despite the daily stress Elaine experienced as a nurse at an obstetrician/gynecologist's office. She had no side effects, and her blood sugar was under control.

But as often happens with medications, the Diabeta eventually stopped working. Her blood glucose began to go up at the end of the day. The doctor suggested she split the pill in two, taking 2.5 mg in the morning and 2.5 mg at night. "But you know when you split a pill, you don't always get the same amount in each half," Elaine says.

When that strategy failed, Elaine's doctor put her on Glucophage XR (metformin). Metformin acts on the liver by limiting the amount of stored glucose it releases and lowering your need for insulin. Metformin also helps reduce blood glucose by making muscles more sensitive to insulin, which promotes the absorption of glucose. In addition, it decreases the amount of sugar that gets absorbed into your intestines.

Glucophage is commonly prescribed to overweight patients like Elaine because the drug is less likely to cause weight gain than some of the other diabetes medications. To help her body become accustomed to it, her doctor eased her into the Glucophage, gradually increasing her dosage to four pills of 500 mg each a day.

Still, Elaine's fasting blood sugars were high, and her doctor decided to add Amaryl (glimepiride), a sulfonylurea, to her regimen. She took Amaryl in the morning and the Glucophage XR at dinner. "It really helped," Elaine says. "My blood sugars were in a normal range, and my A1C was normal, too. But then it almost helped too much."

Elaine began to experience bouts of hypoglycemia that left her feeling shaky, weak, and extremely hungry. "I always know when it's going down," Elaine says. "You feel really shaky, and you have a funny little headache that can quickly turn into a real headache. Sometimes, you feel weak, and you can't walk."

She talked it over with her doctor, who then switched her to Actos, a thiazolidinedione, which works by making your body tissues more sensitive to insulin. Actos also helps inhibit the liver from releasing too much stored glucose.

Using Actos proved to be a disaster. Elaine developed edema, gained weight, and started having a series of upper respiratory infections that she suspects may have been related to the use of Actos. "In the first week, I gained seven pounds of water," she says. "And my feet were so swollen that it hurt to walk."

Worst of all, the drug wasn't even helping to lower her blood glucose. Most mornings, she awoke to a fasting blood sugar of about 194 mg/dl. She then took Actos but only reduced her blood sugar to 184 mg/dl hours later. "I also didn't like worrying about how the drug was going to affect my liver," she says.

Elaine reported the side effects to her doctor, and she went back on the Amaryl. Now, she's back to taking 2 mg of Amaryl in the morning to lower her fasting blood glucose levels. At dinner, she takes 2,000 mg of Glucophage XR. Her fasting blood glucose are still slightly elevated, but are usually normal during the day.

Her blood glucose still dips at times, but it beats the swelling and weight gain that occurred with Actos, Elaine says. She hopes to find out if her doctor will lower her dosage of Amaryl to prevent any episodes of hypoglycemia.

CHAPTER SEVEN 🌿

Short-Term Complications of Diabetes

Having diabetes isn't easy, as you well know by now. But some days, the illness can pose additional complications that can make you sicker than normal. A plummet in blood sugar can trigger hypoglycemia and seizures. A drop in insulin levels may lead to diabetic ketoacidosis. An undetected surge in blood glucose can put you at risk for hyperglycemic hyperosmolar non-ketotic coma (HHNC).

Some diabetics may experience these complications frequently. Others may never have even one complication. Either way, it's important to know the short-term complications that can impact your health and to learn ways to prevent them that will help you avoid any serious long-term effects. You should discuss these potential problems with your health-care team and decide on a strategy in advance.

Hypoglycemia

For many people with diabetes, hypoglycemia, or low blood sugar, is a constant threat. Hypoglycemia usually occurs when blood sugars fall below 50 to 60 mg/dl, but can vary from one person to the next. Several circumstances can trigger hypoglycemia, including:

- Skipping a meal.
- Sleeping later than usual, especially if it's been a long time since you last ate.
- Exercising too strenuously or for too long.
- Sexual activity. People prone to hypoglycemia at night or during exercise may also experience it during sex.
- Taking too much insulin.
- Waiting too long to eat after taking your insulin.
- Drinking alcohol on an empty stomach. When your blood glucose levels drop, your liver usually responds by releasing stored glucose. But if there's alcohol in the blood, your liver becomes more preoccupied with eliminating the alcohol than with releasing glucose. Alcohol also impairs judgment, so you may become less alert to the symptoms of hypoglycemia.
- Some diabetics are prone to having hypoglycemia in the middle of the night, often without their knowing it. But sometimes, there are clues that reveal you've had hypoglycemia, such as dampness in your sheets and pajamas, restless sleep and nightmares, a morning headache or fatigue.

Symptoms

Not every attack of hypoglycemia is life threatening. In fact, if you detect it early on, you can treat it quickly and easily by eating a fast-acting carbohydrate such as fruit juice. But left unchecked, you can develop a severe case of hypoglycemia. The key is recognizing the symptoms.

During a bout of mild hypoglycemia, you may suddenly feel weak and very hungry. You may tremble and shake, and your heartbeat may speed up. You may also experience chills, anxiety, lightheadedness, and nervousness. These symptoms are linked to the autonomic nervous system of the body, which controls the opening of blood vessels, the beating of your heart, and the rate of your breathing. Most people can recognize these symptoms and are able to treat the problem themselves.

In the case of moderate hypoglycemia, the reduction of blood glucose has started to affect the brain. Many of the symptoms are like those for mild hypoglycemia, but you may also have a headache, mood changes, irritability, nausea, blurred vision, numbness in the lips or tongue, confusion, and a decrease in your ability to pay attention.

If the condition is still ignored, you may develop severe hypoglycemia, a potentially life-threatening complication. When your brain has been deprived of glucose for too long, you may have convulsions or lose consciousness. When hypoglycemia becomes severe, you need immediate medical attention.

People who have frequent episodes of hypoglycemia should talk to their doctors about it. Together, you should discuss strategies to prevent hypoglycemia and make sure you know what to do in the event of an emergency.

Who's at Risk

Certain diabetics are more vulnerable to hypoglycemia than others. Anyone who is treating diabetes with intensive therapy is at risk. So are people who have Type 1 diabetes, who may have as many as one or two episodes a week. Other diabetics who use insulin and oral medications are also more susceptible to hypoglycemia. Elderly people have a greater risk for hypoglycemia, too, especially if they have other complications, and/or take insulin or oral medications.

What to Do

The instant you feel hypoglycemia coming on, eat something that contains 10 to 15 mg of carbohydrates. That might be two tablespoons of raisins, two to five glucose tablets, four ounces of soda or fruit juice, five to seven Lifesaver candies, or six jelly beans. Test your blood glucose, if you can. Ideally, it should be higher than 70 mg/dl. If not, try eating another carbohydrate-rich food and testing your blood sugar again in fifteen minutes.

If you're experiencing a case of moderate hypoglycemia, there's a chance your judgment is impaired. You may also be confused and belligerent, even resistant to doing anything to correct the problem. Make sure that people around you know your risk for hypoglycemia and know what to do in this situation. You should try to eat 10 to 15 mg of carbohydrates and test your blood glucose. If it's still low, eat more carbohydrates. An episode of severe hypoglycemia almost always requires medical attention.

When You Need Glucagon

Most people in the midst of a severe hypoglycemic episode will require a shot of glucagon to revive them. Glucagon is a fast-acting hormone made in the pancreas that halts the liver's release of insulin and promotes the release of glucose. Glucagon doesn't work in people who have no glucose stored in the liver, which can happen in people with chronic hypoglycemia or in alcoholics.

Diabetics who are prone to hypoglycemia are generally advised to keep a glucagon kit around, in case of an emergency. The kits are available by prescription. Be sure that you and others around you are familiar with the use of glucagon before an emergency occurs.

Like insulin, glucagon is injected into fatty tissue or muscle. After an injection, you become nauseated or vomit and should keep your head elevated above your stomach. Once you're revived, drink a clear fluid such as ginger ale to settle the stomach and try to eat a substantial snack such as a roll with peanut butter. If you don't respond to the first dose of glucagon, you may require another shot. In the meantime, someone should get medical help.

What Is Hypoglycemia Unawareness?

Although some people are quick to detect the symptoms of hypoglycemia, some people may be completely oblivious, a condition known as hypoglycemia unawareness. These people typically experience impaired judgment in the early stages of hypoglycemia, which makes it difficult for them to notice the symptoms and signs. The problem puts them at risk for an unexpected case of hypoglycemia that quickly becomes severe. The condition is common in people who closely monitor their blood glucose and also in pregnant women. It can also occur in people who have had several episodes of hypoglycemia and stop sensing the signs of it.

If you are prone to hypoglycemia unawareness, you should test your blood glucose more frequently during the day. You should always do a test before driving or exercising. You may also want to consider raising your blood glucose goals to 140 mg/dl instead of 120 mg/dl. Also, be sure to tell people around you that you're prone to hypoglycemia and educate them on how to treat it.

Preventing Hypoglycemia

People who are prone to hypoglycemia might need to take some preventive measures to keep their blood sugar from getting too low. Here are some good ways to keep hypoglycemia at bay:

1. Watch how much you eat and when you eat. Skipping meals or eating less food than you normally do is not a good idea if you get hypoglycemia. You also shouldn't wait too long to eat after an insulin injection.
2. If you feel even a twinge of hypoglycemia during exercise, stop immediately. Always keep a fast-acting carbohydrate-rich food handy, and eat it if you feel any symptoms. If you've had a previous bout of low blood sugar in the past doing the same activity, try eating an extra snack before, during, or after the exercise to stave off another episode.
3. Anticipate low blood glucose if it tends to dip during sex. Eat a snack beforehand or change the timing of your insulin, so it doesn't go into high gear in the heat of passion.

4. Consider eating a bedtime snack if you have nocturnal hypoglycemia. A high-protein snack is especially helpful since protein helps stimulate the production of glucagon. The snack is even more important if you did a lot of physical activity during the day.

5. Develop an insulin strategy so that insulin levels don't peak in the middle of the night. That might mean taking an intermediate-acting insulin at bedtime or programming your pump so it releases less insulin the middle of the night.

6. Always drink alcohol in moderation. In general, women should limit themselves to one drink a day and men to two. One drink is twelve ounces of beer or wine spritzer, five ounces of wine, or 1.5 ounces of 80 proof distilled spirits. Never drink on an empty stomach, which only elevates your risk for hypoglycemia.

7. Test your blood glucose as soon as you wake up, especially if you do sleep in. If necessary, take a fast-acting carbohydrate. If you plan to sleep late, reduce your nighttime dose of long-acting insulin by 10 to 15 percent or eat a little snack at bedtime. Just be sure to check your blood glucose to make sure it's not too high in the morning.

Hyperglycemia

On the opposite end of the spectrum is hyperglycemia, or high blood sugar. As a diabetic, you already have blood glucose that tends to get higher than normal. When you have hyperglycemia, your blood sugar is generally 250 mg/dl or higher.

Hyperglycemia can result from several factors, including:

- Eating too many carbohydrates.
- Skipping your insulin.
- Eating too soon after an insulin injection.
- Using insulin that was expired, or exposed to extreme temperatures.

- Injecting insulin near a mole, scar, or swollen area, which can delay its absorption.
- Faulty functioning of the pump. The needle on a pump may become dislodged, or the infusion line could be detached from the pump, causing insulin to leak out. You may also have dead batteries, kinks, or air in the infusion line, or an empty insulin cartridge. An incorrect setting of your basal rate could also elevate blood glucose.
- Monthly menstrual cycle or menopause.
- Illness, stress, and other changes in your normal routine.
- Some people experience the dawn phenomenon, or the Somogyi effect, high blood glucose upon awakening.

Symptoms

The symptoms of hyperglycemia are just like those of having diabetes. Often, they're subtle or even unnoticeable unless you're closely monitoring your blood glucose. But if you do have symptoms, you may feel tired and lethargic. You may be urinating more frequently than normal, and you may be extremely thirsty.

Having these high levels over a sustained period of time can affect how well your body functions. Ultimately, it can cause severe complications or worsen the ones you already have. The long-term complications of diabetes will be examined more closely in the next chapter.

Who's at Risk

People who rely on insulin are at risk for hyperglycemia. So are people who have undiagnosed or untreated diabetes who may be simply unaware that they have high blood glucose. Left untreated, blood sugars can rise to frightening heights of as much as 1,000 mg/dl.

Complications from Hyperglycemia

Even the most conscientious diabetic will have periods when blood glucose goes up and down. But when blood glucose is high for extended periods, other complications, such as diabetic ketoacidosis and hyper-glycemic hypersomolar non-ketotic coma (HHNC) can quickly develop. These conditions are life-threatening and require immediate medical attention.

Diabetic Ketoacidosis or DKA

Hyperglycemia that goes unnoticed or untreated in Type 1 diabetics can result in diabetic ketoacidosis, also called DKA. This rare, but serious condition is more common in girls, especially among those aged fifteen or under who may abandon their insulin regimen out of embarrassment or shame. Young girls with eating disorders who skip meals or insulin injections are at risk for DKA. The condition is also more likely to occur during periods of stress or illness. Physical and emotional stress causes the body to produce hormones that tell the liver to release stored glucose. In addition, alcoholics are at greater risk for developing DKA.

The onset of DKA begins when the body doesn't have enough insulin to escort the extra glucose to body cells. Your body becomes starved for energy and begins to break down fat and protein to satisfy its energy needs. The breakdown of fats causes a buildup of substances called ketones. As ketones accumulate in your blood, the individual will develop acidosis, a condition in which the blood experiences a decrease in pH and breathing becomes rapid and shallow, a breathing pattern known as Kussmaul's respirations. The hyperglycemia causes the excess glucose to spill into your urine. To remove it, your kidneys start producing more urine, and you wind up dehydrated.

Symptoms of DKA

A telltale warning sign of DKA is a high blood glucose reading of 250 mg/dl or higher. Other symptoms include increased urination, diminished appetite, nausea, stomach pains, vomiting, blurry vision, trouble breathing, feeling flushed, weakness, drowsiness, a fruity odor on your breath, and intense thirst. If you test your urine, you may also notice elevated levels of ketones.

Treating DKA

If your blood glucose is 250 mg/dl or higher and you're experiencing other symptoms, or if your ketone levels are high, call your doctor right away. Chances are, you need to take a fast-acting insulin, but the dosage information should come from your physician. In the meantime, drink plenty of water, and restrict physical activity. Exercise will burn more fat, and counteract the beneficial effects of the extra insulin.

If your high ketone levels are accompanied by uncontrollable vomiting, get medical help right away. You will need insulin therapy from trained emergency personnel to bring your glucose levels under control.

Hospitalization

Twenty percent of all diabetics who are hospitalized wind up there because of DKA. The condition is highly dangerous and can lead to difficulties breathing, shock, coma, and death.

Often, it takes twenty-four to thirty-six hours to treat DKA and bring glucose and ketone levels under control. In addition to insulin, you will receive fluids to replace those you have lost and potassium, salt, and electrolytes to restore balance in your body. Depending on the cause of the DKA episode, its severity, and other complications, you may be kept in the hospital for several days.

Can DKA Be Prevented?

You bet it can! Like many complications associated with diabetes, the key is closely monitoring your blood glucose. Frequent checks will alert you to the first signs of DKA, which is blood glucose above 250 mg/dl. Regular monitoring is also helpful because it allows you to rein in rising blood glucose before it gets out of hand.

And because DKA is caused by insufficient amounts of insulin, it's absolutely critical that you do not skip a dose—ever. Also, carefully monitor the equipment that delivers your insulin. Store your insulin properly, making sure to avoid extreme temperatures. Check to make sure your pump is in good working order.

When you're sick or stressed out, make an extra effort to keep close watch on ketone levels as well. During these times, you should check your blood and urine every four hours if you're at risk for DKA. You should also check your urine for ketones whenever you feel nauseous or are vomiting.

Hyperglycemic Hyperosmolar Non-Ketotic Coma

In some patients with Type 2 diabetes, blood sugar levels can get dangerously high, producing a condition known as hyperglycemic hyperosomolar state (HHS) or hyperglycemic hyperosmolar non-ketotic coma (HHNC). HHNC may occur in patients who don't even know they have diabetes, in which case HHNC becomes the first indication that something is wrong.

The condition begins when blood sugar levels increase. In order to eliminate the excess glucose, your body produces more urine, which in turn causes dehydration. The process may continue for days, even weeks before you're aware of the problem. The constant dehydration eventually begins to impair your thinking. Confusion sets in, and it may become increasingly difficult for you to realize that you need a drink of water or to urinate. The extra glucose causes the blood to thicken, and can result in brain swelling, leading to stupor, coma, or death.

Elderly people, who are less capable of taking care of themselves, are at high risk for HHNC. In fact, elderly people in nursing homes account for a third of all cases of HHNC. Another group at high risk are those with diabetes who have not been diagnosed. They account for another third of all cases. Unaware of the symptoms for diabetes, these people can have blood glucose climb to high levels with little warning.

The condition is also more likely to occur during illness, infection, or periods of stress, when the body produces extra glucose.

In addition, you are at greater risk for HHS if you are on medications that can elevate blood glucose levels, such as cimitedine (Tagamet), glucocorticoids, and beta blockers. Blood glucose levels can also rise if you are receiving peritoneal dialysis or intravenous feedings, which raises your risk. People who abuse alcohol are also at greater risk for HHS since the alcohol restricts the amount of insulin available.

Symptoms
The symptoms of HHS are much more subtle than those for DKA. Be on the lookout for dry, parched mouth, extreme thirst, and sleepiness or confusion. You may also experience warm, dry skin without sweating. If you have any of these symptoms, check your blood glucose immediately. Levels of 350 mg/dl should prompt an immediate call to your doctor. If blood glucose is above 500 mg/dl, get to a hospital as soon as possible or summon emergency help.

Treatment for HHS
Like DKA, the treatment for HHS requires a combination of insulin, fluids, and electrolytes. Since you may lose as much as 15 percent of your total body weight to dehydration, replacing those lost fluids is of utmost importance. For that, you may receive saline solution for several hours until your fluid levels return to normal.

Can HHS Be Prevented?
Your best weapon against HHS is to keep close watch on blood glucose levels. Simply doing a check once or twice a day is enough to alert you to a probable problem. A sudden rise in blood glucose should intensify your vigilance and prompt more frequent checks.

You should also closely monitor your blood glucose during periods of illness and stress, when levels are likely to rise. Doing blood glucose checks as frequently as three or four times a day can help during illness and stress. While you're ill, make sure to get plenty of fluids, but steer clear of alcoholic beverages and those that contain caffeine.

Talk to your medical team about what to do when you do get a high reading of 250 mg/dl or higher. You may require insulin, even if it's not a part of your normal regimen.

Other Complications

Not every short-term complication of diabetes is life-threatening. Some may just be temporary problems that need to be addressed before they become more dangerous.

Dawn Phenomenon

Every morning, in the hours before you awaken, your body begins to secrete growth hormones that suppress the effects of insulin. Without insulin, your blood glucose begins to rise, giving you the energy surge you need to get out of bed and start your day. The steady rise occurs usually between 4 a.m. and 8 a.m. and is a natural part of your body's circadian rhythms.

But in diabetics, it can trigger a bout of high blood glucose called the Dawn Phenomenon. You may awaken extremely thirsty, with a strong need to urinate. Your vision may be blurry. Or you may have no symptoms at all, just a blood glucose reading that is higher than it should be.

Dawn Phenomenon is not a life-threatening complication, but you should discuss it with your doctor, especially if your blood glucose is 200 mg/dl or higher. By itself, Dawn Phenomenon is unlikely to cause a lasting bout of hyperglycemia. But if you don't bring it down, something as simple as eating too much at breakfast could lead to a more serious case of hyperglycemia.

Somogyi Phenomenon

A rapid shift from low to high levels of blood glucose is called the Somogyi phenomenon, or rebound hyperglycemia. It occurs when the body responds to hypoglycemia—oddly enough—with hyper-glycemia. If the initial hypoglycemia is not treated properly, a cycle of hypoglycemia and hyperglycemia can result.

In healthy people, a drop in blood glucose triggers the release of epinephrine, norepinephrine, glucagon, cortisol, and growth hormones that help bring blood glucose back up to normal levels. As the blood glucose rises, insulin is released to help move it out of the bloodstream. In people with diabetes however, the insulin response is limited or absent. Blood glucose remains high. Sometimes, simply eating too much carbohydrate-rich food to counteract hypoglycemia can cause blood glucose to swing high, and bring on the Somogyi phenomenon.

The symptoms of the Somogyi phenomenon are the same as those for hypoglycemia and hyperglycemia. But you may notice only one of those. The only way to know if you're experiencing rebound hyper-glycemia is to take your blood glucose between 2 and 3 a.m. and be on the lookout for a blood glucose below 60 mg/dl.

Is It Dawn or Somogyi?

If waking up to high blood glucose is a frequent morning event, you should try to determine if it's the Dawn phenomenon or the Somogyi phenomenon. The only way to do that is to test blood glucose in the middle of the night, around 3 a.m. If the levels are low at that hour, then it's most likely a case of Somogyi phenomenon. You may need to eat a bedtime snack to counter the effect or lower your evening dose of insulin.

If however, your middle-of-the-night blood glucose is normal or high, then the morning high is most likely the result of the Dawn phenomenon. In this case, your doctor may suggest you increase your dose of insulin at bedtime or shift your dinnertime insulin to a later hour.

Brittle Diabetes

Before blood glucose monitoring became routine, people with diabetes were more susceptible to frequent highs and lows in blood sugar. The condition, known as brittle diabetes, has become less common, now that diabetics can detect these swings in blood glucose, figure out the reasons behind them, and exert greater control over preventing them.

But some people still have these extremes caused by exaggerated responses to food, medications, exercise, and stress. Eating the same food every day at the same time does little to calm these drastic highs and lows, and regular exercise or a rigid regimen of insulin doesn't help either.

The symptoms of brittle diabetes are just like those for hypoglycemia and hyperglycemia. But it's always best to measure your blood glucose to know for sure if it's swinging up and down. Extreme highs or lows can cause unconsciousness, seizures, coma, and death. In the long-term, frequent swings in blood glucose can raise your risk for serious complications of diabetes, such as retinopathy, kidney disease, heart disease, and infections.

If you are prone to brittle diabetes, consult your medical team about what to do when it occurs. One way to treat this condition is by using a seventy-two hour glucose monitoring system, which will continuously measure your blood glucose for up to three days, in conjunction with an insulin pump. The constant measuring will let you anticipate dips and rises in blood glucose, while the pump will allow you to adjust your insulin accordingly.

Of course, preventing brittle diabetes in the first place is ideal. To do that, you must find the reasons behind the swings in blood glucose. Be on the lookout for possible causes including:

- *The timing of your insulin injections.* You need thirty to forty-five minutes for your regular insulin to start working before you eat. With the new short-acting insulin analogs such as Humalog and Novolog, one should eat within five to ten minutes of taking your insulin. When in doubt, take the insulin analog at the time the meal is served to prevent hypoglycemia.
- *The accuracy of your insulin doses.* Too much insulin at one time may go to work in varying intervals.

- *The depth of your injection.* Inject your insulin at the same depth every time.
- *Injecting insulin in extreme temperatures.* If your body is warm, it will speed up the rate that insulin is absorbed. If you're in a cool environment, it could slow it down.
- *Dehydration.* If high blood glucose has caused you to become dehydrated, you may have a hard time absorbing insulin.

Prevent and Prepare

The best course of action in dealing with any short-term complication is prevention. That's why frequent blood glucose checks are so critical. By keeping an eye on how high or low your blood glucose is, you can be on the lookout for changes that signal impending problems.

But as a diabetic, you should also be prepared for a medical emergency. Even if you are diligent about checking your blood glucose, there may be days when you eat the wrong amount of food, don't inject your insulin just right or forget to take an oral medication. Talk to your medical team about what to do in the event of any emergency. Wear a bracelet that identifies you as a diabetic, so strangers know to summon medical help. Educate your friends and family about what to do in the event of an emergency. Knowing what to do in advance will help you survive an unexpected medical crisis and limit the impact it can have on your health and well-being.

CHAPTER EIGHT 🌿

Cardiovascular Complications

Diabetes can have dire, even deadly, consequences for your heart. Cardiovascular disease is the leading cause of premature death among people with diabetes, with at least 65 percent of all diabetics dying from heart disease or stroke. Both conditions are the result of cardiovascular disease (CVD). In fact, according to a 2002 survey by the American Diabetes Association, physicians said they believe that diabetes poses a greater risk for cardiovascular disease than any other factor, including smoking, high blood pressure, high cholesterol, or obesity.

Why is CVD so prevalent among diabetics? Because the people who are likely to develop diabetes are also likely to have high blood pressure and high cholesterol, and to be overweight or obese. Together they can add up to a lethal combination. Consider these grim statistics:

- People with diabetes are two to four times more likely to have heart disease or suffer a stroke than people without diabetes.
- A person with Type 2 diabetes has the same risk for heart attack as someone without diabetes who already had a heart attack.

- People with diabetes are more likely to die from a heart attack and are more likely than healthy people to have a second heart attack.
- Adults younger than 45 who have Type 2 diabetes are fourteen times more likely to have a heart attack and thirty times more likely to have a stroke than nondiabetic peers.

What Is Cardiovascular Disease?

The term cardiovascular disease refers to a broad category of diseases that are linked to how efficiently your heart pumps blood (cardio) or how well your blood circulates through your blood vessels (vascular). It is not a single disorder or condition, but rather a collection of diseases that affect any part of your cardiovascular system.

The two diseases you should know about are:

- *Atherosclerosis.* When cholesterol and other fatty substances collect on the walls of your arteries, they form yellow deposits called atheroma that cause the arteries to narrow. Once narrowed, blood no longer flows smoothly through your arteries. The muscle layer of the artery thickens, and the narrowing worsens.

   Blood platelets that are responsible for clotting may start to collect in clumps on the surface of the deposits, creating dangerous blood clots that can interfere even further with blood flow. If a clot grows large, it may completely block the artery and cut off blood supply to an organ.

   Atherosclerosis produces no symptoms. Often, it isn't until a heart attack or stroke occurs that patients even know their arteries are hardening and narrowing. The condition is a direct result of too much cholesterol in the blood, which is typically elevated in people who have diabetes. Smoking, lack of regular exercise, being overweight, and high blood pressure also contribute to the development of atherosclerosis.

• *Coronary artery disease (CAD).* If atherosclerosis occurs in an artery leading to the heart, the result is coronary artery disease. Without enough blood flowing to the heart, the heart muscle gets damaged. Although there may be no symptoms initially, later on, you may develop angina, a pain in the chest that occurs with exertion. In some people, CAD can cause arrhythmias, or abnormal heart rhythms, that can bring on palpitations, light-headedness, or fainting. Older people who develop CAD may get chronic heart failure, in which the heart becomes too weak to pump enough blood through the body.

Progression of Atherosclerosis and CAD

Many people don't know they have atherosclerosis or CAD. But if you have diabetes, your risk for both conditions goes up and substantially increases the chance that you could have a heart attack or stroke.

• Heart attack, also called myocardial infarction, occurs when the blood supply to the heart muscle is severely reduced or stopped. The cutoff of blood flow is the result of a blockage in one of the coronary arteries that supplies blood to the heart. The blockage comes from atherosclerosis, the buildup of plaque, or fatty deposits, on artery walls. Eventually, the plaque bursts, tears, or ruptures, causing a blood clot to form. Once it's fully formed, the clot interrupts blood flow, causing the heart attack. If the blood supply is cut off for more than a few minutes, the heart muscle cells can suffer permanent damage and die. Depending on the extent of the damage, a heart attack can cause death.

• Stroke occurs when the blood supply to the brain is cut off. Like heart attack, the roots of a stroke start with the buildup of fatty deposits on artery walls. The fatty deposits may form a blood clot in the clogged part of the blood vessel: This is called cerebral thrombosis, and it can cause a stroke. Most strokes are the result of cerebral thrombosis. A stroke can also occur if a clot forms elsewhere in the circulatory system and travels to the blood vessels leading to the brain, a process called cerebral embolism. A hemorrhagic stroke, which is less common, results from the rupturing of a weakened blood vessel.

Some people may experience transient ischemic attacks (TIAs), brief episodes in which the brain ceases functioning because of a temporary deprivation of oxygen due to blocked blood vessels. Symptoms of a TIA are slurred speech, weakness of an arm or leg, weakness of the face, or double vision. If a TIA lasts longer than an hour, the event is called a stroke. Without treatment, a person who has a TIA is more likely to have a stroke later on.

Why Is Diabetes a Risk Factor?

Every day, our hearts work hard to send blood along 60,000 miles of blood vessels throughout our bodies, nourishing cells with nutrients, glucose, oxygen, and other substances that help you stay alive. In healthy people, the blood flows smoothly. But in a person with diabetes, blood flow can be compromised and disrupted by the extra glucose that is also in circulation.

Excess glucose affects the quality of your blood in several ways:

- *It changes the amount and makeup of the lipoproteins in your blood.* These lipoproteins transport fats to your body cells. If there's too much fat and cholesterol in your blood vessels, these substances will stick to your artery walls, causing atherosclerosis, a narrowing and thickening of the vessels.
- *It makes the cholesterol and fat circulating in your blood stickier.* The stickier these substances become, the more likely they are to adhere to blood vessel walls.

- *It can release a substance in your blood platelets that will make them more prone to clotting.* A higher risk of clotting will increase the likelihood that artery walls will narrow.

If the arteries that supply the heart are narrowed, you develop coronary artery disease. If blood to a portion of the heart is cut off, you have a heart attack or myocardial infarction. If blood cannot reach the brain, you have a stroke.

People with Type 2 diabetes face a greater risk for cardiovascular disease than their healthy peers because most patients are also prone to high blood pressure, high cholesterol, and obesity. Taken together, all these factors raise the odds for developing heart disease.

Other Risk Factors

Not every person who has diabetes will develop cardiovascular disease, or have a heart attack or stroke. But the risk definitely increases if certain other conditions are present. Often, these conditions coexist with diabetes. They are:

High Blood Pressure

Like diabetes, high blood pressure, or hypertension, is a silent condition, providing no clues that anything is even wrong. Often, it isn't until you are diagnosed with something else, such as heart disease or diabetes, that you learn you have high blood pressure. As many as 70 percent of all people with diabetes also have high blood pressure.

Blood pressure is the force exerted on the arteries by blood as it circulates through the body. Healthy blood pressure is generally considered anything below 140/90 mmHG. The top number is the systolic pressure; the peak pressure at the moment your heart contracts and pumps blood. The bottom number, known as diastolic pressure, is the level of pressure that occurs when your heart relaxes to let blood flow into your heart. The higher your blood pressure, the harder your heart is working to pump blood throughout your body. Over time, the added stress can damage your arteries, causing them to narrow and clog.

Having both diabetes and hypertension worsens your risk for cardiovascular disease because both conditions can damage the arteries. Together, they greatly increase your odds for having a heart attack or stroke. Fortunately, many of the same lifestyle recommendations to treat high blood pressure are the same ones for heart disease, such as losing weight by getting more exercise and eating a healthy diet.

High Cholesterol

Another common problem for diabetics is high cholesterol. Cholesterol is a fat-like substance that your liver produces naturally and that you get from the foods you eat. Inside the body, cholesterol has several vital functions such as synthesizing vitamin D in the skin, aiding in the digestion of fats, and helping in the production of important hormones such as estrogen, testosterone, and cortisol. Too much cholesterol, however, can contribute to the hardening of your arteries.

Cholesterol is not just one single substance but actually several components, which are measured on what is known as a lipid profile. The ones you should know are:

- *High-density lipoproteins,* or HDLs, known as the good cholesterol. These are the lipoproteins that carry cholesterol out of the blood and into the liver, where it is broken down and eliminated from the body. Women who have diabetes should try to have a total of 55 mg/dl, while men should aim for 45 mg/dl.
- *Low density lipoproteins,* or LDLs, known as the bad or harmful cholesterol. These lipoproteins have the dubious distinction of transporting cholesterol into your body cells. Having too much LDL will cause the cholesterol to stick to artery walls, causing the buildup of plaque that hardens and narrows blood vessels. In people with diabetes, LDL particles are generally smaller

and more damaging than they are in healthy people. Diabetics should keep LDLs at 100 mg/dl or less. If you have had an angioplasty or heart attack, the LDL cholesterol should be less than 80 mg/dl.

- *Triglycerides.* Most of the stored fat in your body is in the form of triglycerides. When your body needs them, the liver and fat cells release triglycerides to meet your energy needs. Too many triglycerides however, raise your risk for heart disease. Triglycerides are transported in the body by very-low density lipoproteins (VLDL), which may be measured on a lipid profile. Triglycerides are 20 percent VLDL cholesterol. People with diabetes should have triglycerides below 150 mg/dl.
- *Total cholesterol* is just as the name suggests: the total amount of cholesterol you have in your blood, or LDL + HDL + VLDL. Ideally, people who have diabetes should aim for a total cholesterol of 200 mg/dl or less. If HDL is high, you may have a total cholesterol that is elevated and still be in great shape. Ideally, the total cholesterol divided by HDL cholesterol should be less than five. If it is greater than five, you have a higher risk of developing CVD.

Some diabetics develop diabetic dyslipidemia, also called atherogenic dyslipidemia. The condition is associated with insulin resistance and is marked by high levels of triglycerides, high levels of small LDL particles, and low levels of HDL.

Obesity

There's no doubt about it: the epidemic of obesity in this country is directly connected to the rising number of people who are being diagnosed with diabetes. According to the Centers for Disease Control and Prevention, the number of obese Americans has gone up 74 percent between 1991 and 2001. In that same period, the number of

Americans diagnosed with diabetes increased 61 percent. Coincidence? Highly unlikely.

Experts agree that being obese and overweight are major risk factors for cardiovascular disease. The unhealthy diets and lack of activity that made you overweight also promote the development of cardiovascular disease that damages the arteries. Obesity is also a risk factor for having Type 2 diabetes. Fatty tissue is generally more resistant to the effects of insulin, and heavy people have more of it. Approximately 80 percent of all cases of Type 2 diabetes in the U.S. occur in people who are overweight or obese.

Age and Race
Certain ethnic groups are at greater risk for diabetes and its complications. They include African Americans, Hispanic/Latino Americans, American Indians, Asian Americans, and Pacific Islanders. The incidence of diabetic complications also increases with age.

Metabolic Syndrome
A combination of these factors has been identified as another risk for developing heart disease, known as metabolic syndrome. The National Cholesterol Education Program (NCEP) recently presented risk factors for heart disease and heart disease equivalents called the ATP III guidelines. A person who has metabolic syndrome may have:

- A waistline of more than forty inches in men and thirty-five inches in women.
- Blood glucose levels above 109. (New ADA guidelines have set blood glucose levels above 100 as pre-diabetic.)
- A systolic blood pressure above 130 and a diastolic blood pressure above 85.
- Triglyceride level above 200.
- HDL cholesterol below 40 in men and 50 in women.
- LDL above 100.

Each factor counts as one and people who have any three are said to have metabolic syndrome. According to the Third National Health and Nutrition Examination Survey (NHANES III), approximately 44 percent of the U.S. population over age fifty has metabolic syndrome. The research found that people who have both diabetes and metabolic syndrome had the highest prevalence of coronary heart disease (CHD) with 19.2 percent affected. Of those people who had metabolic syndrome without diabetes, 13.9 percent had CHD.

The bottom line is this: The combination of obesity and mild blood glucose elevations can cause even moderate insulin resistance and raise your risk for coronary heart disease. People who have these risk factors should be treated as if they have diabetes and told to lose weight, exercise, and eat a healthy diet. The condition can even occur in children and young adults. A concerted prevention plan could benefit everyone in the family and lower the risk for heart disease.

How Do I Know If I Have CVD?

Truth is, you don't always know. The symptoms of cardiovascular disease vary greatly among individuals and depend on the type of specific disease you have.

Some people may experience angina, a pain in the center of the chest that feels like squeezing, burning, or aching. Angina occurs when the heart isn't getting as much blood and oxygen as it needs. You may feel short of breath or have pressure and tightness in the chest, or pain in the chest that radiates down the inside of the left arm while you're climbing stairs, lugging heavy packages, having sex, or doing exercise.

For some patients, the pain is mild and sporadic, while in others, it may be more pronounced and persistent. Although angina is not a cause of long-term damage to the heart, it is a sign of heart disease.

Other signs of heart disease include shortness of breath, chest pain, and palpitations. You may also have fainting spells that cause you to lose consciousness, edema, fatigue, and a bluish hue in your skin.

If you have any of these signs or symptoms, be sure to bring them to your doctor's attention, especially if you also have high blood pressure or high cholesterol and are overweight. Your physician may order an echocardiogram, stress test (treadmill), or other diagnostic exam to determine whether you have a more serious form of cardiovascular disease.

Your doctor may also use a screening test known as the electron-beam CAT Scan or Ultrafast CAT Scan to determine the extent of damage to your arteries. The test looks at the amount of calcium buildup near the heart and can assess the amount of heart disease you have. The test, which costs about $500 to $600, is frequently not covered by insurance, but may be valuable in determining the amount of heart disease present.

How Do I Know if It's a Heart Attack?

In the movies, a heart attack is sudden and swift. The stricken patient clutches his chest and drops to the ground. But in reality, the process may be considerably slower. It may begin with mild pain or discomfort. You may be unsure what is wrong. But then the pressure on your chest persists, lasting longer than just a few minutes, and starts to spread to the shoulders, neck, and arms. The pain may be accompanied by light-headedness, fainting, sweating, or nausea. Less common symptoms are stomach or abdominal pain, nausea, dizziness, difficulty breathing, inexplicable anxiety, weakness or fatigue, a cold sweat, or palpitations.

Some people with diabetes may feel sick to their stomach or have shortness of breath, but with no chest pain. Other patients may have no indications at all that they're having a heart attack. Or, they may attribute the signs and symptoms to other ailments. A heart attack for instance, may resemble a panic attack, angina, chest pains, maybe even symptoms similar to indigestion. Unfortunately, the uncertainty may cause a delay in seeking prompt medical treatment that can reduce the disability caused by a heart attack and prevent death.

How Do I Know if It's a Stroke?

Like a heart attack, a stroke can come on suddenly with no warning. You may experience weakness or numbness in your face, arm or leg, especially on just one side of your body. You may also develop confusion and difficulty speaking or understanding what others are saying. Some patients have trouble seeing and difficulties with balance and coordination. You may also experience sudden, severe headaches that come from nowhere.

Can I Prevent CVD?

Because so many people with diabetes also have high blood pressure and high cholesterol and are overweight or obese, it may seem virtually impossible for a diabetic to avoid heart disease, especially if your arteries have already started to narrow. But that is entirely untrue. There are strategies you can use to help lower your risk for developing cardiovascular disease and thereby lower your chances of having a heart attack or stroke.

Here's what you can do:

- *Get your blood glucose under control.* Keeping close tabs on your blood glucose every day, throughout the day, can help you bring your blood glucose into the normal range.
- *Quit smoking.* Cigarettes damage the circulatory system by narrowing the blood vessels, causing cells to die.
- *Eat a diet rich in high-fiber foods and low in saturated fat.* Fiber works to help eliminate unhealthy cholesterol from the bloodstream. Reducing your intake of saturated fat can help minimize the buildup of atherosclerotic plaque.
- *Try to lower your blood pressure.* High blood pressure indicates your heart is working too hard. Over time, the exertion exhausts the heart muscle, making it harder to pump blood. Eating less salt, exercising, and avoiding stress can all help lower blood pressure.

- *Exercise regularly.* Physical activity lowers cholesterol and blood pressure, and helps improve insulin resistance.
- *Lose weight.* Carrying excess weight taxes the heart and also puts you at risk for high blood pressure, high cholesterol, and complications from diabetes.
- *Talk to your doctor about taking a daily aspirin.* Research suggests that taking an aspirin every day can lower the risk for cardiac events and is just as effective in the prevention of heart disease in diabetics as it is in non-diabetics.

If You Already Have CVD

Aggressive treatment of cardiovascular disease is critical for patients with diabetes. Your physician may suggest you improve your diet, get more exercise, and lose weight. But sometimes lifestyle changes are not enough to keep cardiovascular risks at bay. In that case, your physician may also prescribe medications that help lower cholesterol and blood pressure. Cardiovascular problems may be treated with any of several medications:

- *Aspirin* acts as a blood thinner. It works to inhibit clotting and prevent blockages in the artery.
- *Beta blockers* help calm the overexerted heart by preventing the action of stress-inducing chemicals such as adrenaline. By doing so, they slow the heart rate, lower blood pressure, and lighten the workload for your heart.
- *Calcium-channel blockers* interfere with the uptake of calcium into the heart muscle and blood vessels. These medications help slow the heart's contractions, relax and dilate the blood vessels, and ultimately lower blood pressure and prevent arrhythmias.
- *Nitrates,* also called vasodilators, are often given after a heart attack and work by dilating the arteries in the heart and veins bringing blood to the heart. The effect is lower blood pressure and a reduction in the heart's demand for oxygen.

- *Statins* are cholesterol-lowering medications that block an enzyme primarily in the liver known as HMG CoA reductase. These are especially effective at lowering LDL cholesterol. Statins may be prescribed in conjunction with a new kind of medication that blocks the uptake of LDL cholesterol in the intestine. Ezetimibe (Zetia) is the first drug of its kind and inhibits the transport of fats and LDL cholesterol. This drug may be used in combination with a statin if you have not achieved your cholesterol goal; or it can be used alone, if you have side effects from statins.
- *Niacin* or nicotinic acid compounds are often used to increase HDL cholesterol. But in diabetics, these medications may increase insulin resistance and in rare cases may cause diabetic ketoacidosis. They should be used with extreme caution in people who have Type 2 diabetes.
- *ACE* (angiotensin-converting enzyme) inhibitors relax the blood vessels that lead directly from the heart by blocking hormones that narrow blood vessels. They help reduce the workload on the heart and improve blood flow.
- *ARBs,* or angiotension receptor blockers, protect against the actions of angiotension II, which causes blood vessels to constrict. ARBs relax and widen the blood vessels, and help to improve blood flow.

Talk to your doctor about treating high cholesterol and high blood pressure with medications. Your physician can help you decide which treatment, if necessary, is best suited for your lifestyle and medical profile.

Do I Need Surgery?
Sometimes, it's too late to undo the damage in your blood vessels. You may already have had a heart attack or stroke. In that case, you may

require surgery to reverse or slow the effects of cardiovascular disease. Some common surgeries include:

- *Laser surgery.* Using a beam of light, a surgeon melts away the blockage that is clogging the artery. This procedure is usually done on minor blockages.
- *Coronary angioplasty.* A catheter with an inflated balloon at the tip is inserted into the narrowed or blocked artery. Once inside, the balloon is inflated, so that it presses against the walls of the artery. The catheter is then removed. In some cases, a stent is inserted to keep the artery propped open.
- *Coronary Artery Bypass Graft.* According to a study called the Bypass Angioplasty Revascularization Investigation, diabetic patients who had a heart attack were more likely to survive five years later if they had bypass surgery than those who had angioplasty. When blockages in the arteries are severe, a surgeon may create a detour around the restricted artery by removing part of a blood vessel from elsewhere in the body. The vessel is then grafted above and below the affected artery, creating a bypass around the detour and allowing blood to flow.

What You Can Do Now

If you are at risk for cardiovascular disease, talk it over with your physician. He may suggest you get an echocardiogram, coronary angiogram, a stress test, or another diagnostic exam to determine the condition of your heart and blood vessels. If necessary, you may be given medications to reduce your risk or surgery to reverse existing damage.

As a diabetic, the most important thing you can do to avoid the complications from cardiovascular disease is to keep blood glucose levels in the normal range, lose weight, and lower your blood pressure and cholesterol levels. You should also stop smoking. Smoking increases blood pressure, promotes platelet clotting, and decreases the oxygen-carrying capacity of red blood cells. Peripheral vascular disease and amputations are also complications of CVD and are almost always associated with smoking. By reducing the impact of these risk factors, you can lower your risk for having cardiovascular disease.

CHAPTER NINE

Other Long-Term Complications

The rigors of having diabetes can be tough and exhausting. Keeping an eye on your blood glucose levels becomes a part of your daily routine. Watching your carbohydrate intake is critical at every meal. Exercise is a necessity, not a luxury. And if you're told to take insulin and medications, giving yourself shots and popping pills also becomes a part of your daily life.

The glucose that gets in your blood from the food you eat is meant to be used up for energy, not to linger in your bloodstream. When it swims in your blood, the glucose can do damage throughout your body. It speeds up the hardening of your arteries that occurs with age, clogs up the blood vessels that nourish your eyes and kidneys, reduces blood flow to the heart and brain, damages nerve cells, and reduces the functioning of your immune system.

The goods news is, having diabetes does not mean you will definitely develop a complication. If you monitor your blood glucose levels closely and keep them as close to normal as possible, you can avoid these complications or at least lower your risk. The Diabetes Control and Complications Trial found that people who do that generally have less damage to the eyes, kidneys, and nerves.

Your family history will also play a role in determining your risk for complications. If your family has a history of high blood pressure, cardiovascular disease, and obesity, then you are at greater risk for complications from diabetes.

For people who have already developed these other conditions, the key remains keeping blood glucose levels as close to normal as possible. That means eating a healthy, well-balanced diet, exercising regularly, and taking your insulin or oral medications. By improving blood glucose control, you can limit the damage from these complications, if they do arise.

Still, every person with diabetes should be familiar with the problems that diabetes can cause and be on the lookout for symptoms. Early detection means early treatment, which can help minimize the damage caused by these complications.

Diabetic Retinopathy

In the back of your eye is the retina, where the images you see are projected. In people who have diabetes, the retina can be damaged, causing a condition known as diabetic retinopathy. The excess glucose damages the blood vessels that supply blood to the retina.

Early on, you may have non-proliferative or background retinopathy, in which the blood vessels can close off or weaken. Once closed or weakened, the vessels leak blood, fluid, or fat into the retina of the eye. Your retina no longer gets all the oxygen and nutrients it needs to function, and your vision may become blurred.

If non-proliferative retinopathy goes untreated and becomes moderate or severe, it can become a more serious condition known as proliferative retinopathy. In this type of retinopathy, the blood deprivation causes new blood vessels to form in the retina. Rather than provide the oxygenated blood and nutrients the retina needs, these new vessels proliferate and grow out of control. Heavy lifting can cause the vessels to rupture. Even rapid eye movement during REM sleep may be associated with bleeding if the proliferative retinopathy goes untreated. When the vessels rupture, blood can leak into the part of the eye in front of the retina, thereby blocking light from entering the eye and impairing vision. Sometimes, the condition will produce scar tissue on the retina. If the scar tissue shrinks, it can tear apart the layers of the retina and cause it to separate from the eye. Ultimately, it can lead to blindness.

During either stage of retinopathy, you may develop macular edema, swelling in the macular, the part of your eye that allows you to see fine detail. Swelling can interfere with your ability to see and cause blindness.

Diabetic retinopathy is more prevalent among Type 1 diabetics, though people who have Type 2 diabetes can also develop it. Type 1 diabetics, who have had diabetes for fifteen years, have a 75 percent chance of developing retinopathy. Among Type 2 diabetics who have had diabetes for fifteen years, as many as 85 percent of all patients have retinopathy. Improved blood sugar control may help delay the onset of this complication. If the HbA1C is kept below 6.5 percent, you may be able to prevent it entirely.

Do I Have Retinopathy?

In the early stages of diabetic retinopathy, there may be no symptoms that anything is wrong. As non-proliferative retinopathy progresses, you may develop blurry vision or distortions in your eyesight. But the only way to know you have it is with an eye exam by an ophthalmologist.

Proliferative retinopathy is more evident. You may notice blurring, floating spots and distortions in your eyesight. You may even experience some loss of vision. If you have macular edema, you may notice distortions or warping of straight lines. If your retina becomes detached, you may notice that your vision is blocked by what resembles a window shade.

Treating Diabetic Retinopathy

Fortunately, diabetic retinopathy can be treated. The most common method of treatment is laser therapy. With focal laser therapy, your ophthalmologist will aim a laser-beam light at the specific sites of your eye that need to be treated. The light can destroy the abnormal blood vessels that don't belong in your eye, fix the ones that are leaking, and inhibit the growth factors that are causing new vessels to grow. Usually, it takes one or two sessions to do focal laser therapy.

Another approach to treatment with laser therapy is panretinal photocoagulation, which is preferred if there are abnormal blood vessels growing on the surface of the optic nerve. Instead of focusing on specific sites, a scattered laser beam is emitted to the damaged regions throughout the retina. Photocoagulation usually requires two or three sessions.

In patients who are experiencing hemorrhaging, retinopathy may be treated with cryotherapy or vitrectomy. Cryotherapy freezes a part of the retina in order to destroy abnormal blood vessel growth. It is often used in patients who had no success with laser therapy.

If the retina is detached, and there's been bleeding in the vitreous humor, you may require a surgery called vitrectomy. During a vitrectomy, the vitreous cavity of the eye is cleared of vitreous gel and blood, and replaced with a clear fluid. Surgery to reattach the retina can then be performed, and laser therapy may be used to repair the retina.

If You Have Macular Edema
Having diabetic retinopathy puts you at risk for macular edema, which can occur at any stage of the retinopathy. Macular edema occurs when fluid leaking from the cells of the retina causes the tissue in the macula to swell. When the macular of the eye swells, you are at risk for losing your vision. You may notice blurring in both your near and far vision, a distortion of straight lines, and a diminished capacity for seeing blue and yellow colors.

If you have any of these symptoms, consult your ophthalmologist immediately. Your ophthalmologist can perform special tests to determine whether you have macular edema. Using angiography or sonography, your doctor can determine where the leaks are coming from and apply focal laser therapy to seal these up and reduce swelling in your macula.

Preventing Retinopathy

Like most problems with diabetes, retinopathy and macular edema are best avoided by keeping blood glucose in the normal range. Controlling your blood sugar in the early stages of retinopathy can reverse non-proliferative retinopathy. If it progresses to proliferative retinopathy, you can limit the damage by keeping control of your blood glucose.

Other Eye Problems in Diabetics

Having diabetes puts you at risk for developing other eye problems. Among them:

- Blurry vision may develop if blood glucose levels are out of control.
- Double vision in diabetics, also called diplopia, can happen if the blood vessels and nerves controlling the movement of your eyes are damaged.
- Cataracts may occur when the lenses of your eyes become cloudy. The condition usually develops in older people, but may set in at an earlier age if you have the disease.
- Glaucoma is a condition in which the pressure from the fluid in your eye is too high. Over time, the high pressure can damage the optic nerve. In diabetics, the problem arises when abnormal blood vessel growth interferes with fluid drainage in the eye, causing it to build up.

Neuropathy

Think of your nervous system as a collection of electrical wires and impulses, activated by your brain, which acts as the control center.

Everything you do, from breathing to taking a drink of water to think-ing, is carried out by the signals sent from your brain to your nerves. When you have diabetes, those nerves, or electrical wires, can become damaged and frayed, causing your nerves to misfire and malfunction. When damage to your nerves occurs, it's called neuropathy.

Although diabetes doesn't usually impair the brain and spinal cord, it does affect all the nerves in your body. Signals may be misfired at the wrong time, or they may not be sent at all. The result may be troubles with bladder control, sexual impotence or dysfunction, weakness in your muscles, or pain in your feet or hands.

Neuropathy, experts believe, is due to damage to the Schwann cells which produce myelin, the coating around nerves. High glucose levels cause the Schwann cells to produce more sorbitol, an alcohol sugar, which causes toxic effects on the cells and cell death. When it occurs, neuropathy is rarely reversible. Basically, there are three types of neuropathy.

Mononeuropathy, or Focal Neuropathy

Damage to a single nerve or group of nerves is called mononeuropathy. When a blood vessel that supplies a nerve is shut off, you may develop focal neuropathy in that nerve. There are several kinds of mononeu-ropathies. Cranial neuropathy affects a single nerve from the brain. Plexopathy may affect nerves to the arms and legs. Radiculopathy in-volves the nerves in the trunk of the body.

You may also be prone to what are called entrapment neuro-pathies. One example is carpal tunnel syndrome, which is more com-mon among people with diabetes than the general population. The condition occurs when the median nerve of the forearm gets squeezed in its tunnel by the carpal bones of the wrists. Carpal tunnel syndrome usually causes pain, tingling, and burning. You may also be prone to dropping things.

Symptoms of some mononeuropathies may resemble more serious complications, such as heart attack or stroke. But most mononeuropathies are not permanent and will go away within six to eight weeks once normal blood glucose levels are achieved.

Peripheral Neuropathy, or Distal Symmetric Polyneuropathy

When the nerves in your peripheral nervous system are affected, you develop peripheral neuropathy. This type of neuropathy is caused by the overproduction of sorbitol in the Schwann cell described earlier. This form of neuropathy may strike nerves in several parts of your body, including the arms, hands, legs, and feet.

The symptoms you experience depend on the nerves that are affected. If the small sensory nerves are involved, you may feel tingling, burning, numbness, or a loss of feeling in your hands or feet. Early symptoms usually appear at night when you put your legs and feet up to go to sleep. They often last thirty to forty minutes before the symptoms go away. If the large sensory nerves are involved, you may have trouble with balance or detecting the position of your feet and toes, which may lead to open sores on your feet or deformities in your toes or feet. In the feet, fractures without pain may lead to a crippling condition called Charcot's joints, in which the small bones of the foot disintegrate, ultimately causing deformity. If the neuropathy attacks the motor nerves that control your muscles, you could lose muscle tone in your hands and feet, and have difficulty getting out of a chair or walking. Motor neuropathies are totally reversible with good control of your diabetes.

The most serious form of neuropathy is the loss of sensation, especially if it occurs in your feet. Without the necessary pain signals, you could subject your feet to injuries that could lead to ulcers, gangrene, and amputation.

Autonomic Neuropathy

Breathing. Digestion. Heartbeat. All these processes are governed by the autonomic nervous system that enables your body to hum along like a well-oiled machine. The autonomic nervous system sends messages from the brain to the internal organs, telling them to do what they need to do to keep your body functioning. When it malfunctions, you can experience all kinds of problems with your internal organs and bodily functions.

- *The stomach and intestines.* Normal digestive processes may slow down, and it may take longer for your intestines to empty. The result may be gastroparesis, or delayed stomach emptying, which can cause nausea, vomiting, constipation, and diarrhea.
- *The bladder.* If you develop neurogenic bladder, your bladder muscles weaken, making it difficult for you to sense when it's full or to completely eliminate the urine in your bladder. The excess urine that isn't eliminated puts you at risk for urinary tract infections.
- *Blood pressure.* When nerves that control your heart rate are out of whack, you may experience abnormal rises and falls in blood pressure. You may feel lightheaded when you stand up.
- *Heart rate.* If the nerves to your heart don't know to slow or speed up at the right times, your heart rate may not respond appropriately. At rest, you may have a racing heart. After exercise, your heart rate may remain abnormally high.
- *Silent heart attack.* If damage to the nerves of your heart is severe, you may receive no indication that you're having a heart attack.
- *Sweating.* Damage to the nerves in your skin can cause you to produce too much or too little sweat. Your skin may also become extremely dry.
- *Sexual dysfunction.* In men, there may be difficulty achieving an erection, while in women, orgasm may be more difficult (see Chapter Ten).

Treating Neuropathy

The way you treat your neuropathy will of course, depend on where it strikes. Some types of neuropathy, such as the autonomic ones affecting the heart, have limited options for treatment. But you can employ preventive strategies like standing up more slowly and increasing your salt intake to raise your blood pressure and prevent lightheadedness.

Other kinds of neuropathy can be treated with medication or surgery. For example, antidepressants and anticonvulsants can help alleviate the pain involved in polyneuropathy. In extreme cases of carpal tunnel syndrome, surgery may help to relieve the pressure and pain.

In many cases, you may find pain relief by bringing blood glucose levels into the normal range, so consider ways you can tighten up glucose control. Keeping blood glucose in a healthy range may help some symptoms disappear altogether. In addition, you should give up smoking and drinking alcohol, both habits that can cause nerve damage. Also be on the lookout for other factors that can worsen neuropathy, such as vitamin B12 deficiency and hypothyroidism. The key to relieving your neuropathy is to openly discuss your symptoms with your physician. Together, you can devise a strategy for relief.

Kidney Disease

The kidneys are your body's hard working filtering system, where toxins enter through tiny blood vessels called capillaries, are converted into urine, and then promptly eliminated. In people with diabetes, these tiny blood vessels become blocked and can no longer filter out the bad stuff in your blood. They also become leaky. Waste products that should have been eliminated wind up remaining in the blood, while good, vital nutrients like protein are lost in the urine.

Diabetes takes a direct toll on the kidneys in 30 to 40 percent of diabetics. Early on, the kidneys go into overdrive to remove the extra blood glucose. When this process goes on for a long period of time, the kidneys are taxed and eventually begin to fail. Often, it isn't until you reach the end stages that you may even notice kidney damage. Instead, you need to rely on medical tests to determine whether you are having problems.

Not all diabetics develop kidney problems, though Type 2 diabetics may have excess protein in the urine at the time of diagnosis. In the early stages, most diabetics also have hyperfiltration, in which the kidneys are working harder than usual. Your doctor can do urine tests that will help you detect hyperfiltration and proteins. But it's the other conditions listed below that you will want to avoid if you want to prevent kidney damage from progressing.

Microalbuminuria

The first sign of kidney disease is microalbuminuria, small amounts of protein in the urine. A routine urine test is the only way to know if you have microalbuminuria. The condition is usually present in Type 2 diabetics at the time of diagnosis and eventually develops in Type 1 diabetics.

The condition signals that there are changes occurring in the blood vessels of your kidneys. Blood vessels that have been damaged by the effects of too much blood glucose typically leak protein into the urine. The problem is made worse if you also have high blood pressure, especially if you have Type 2 diabetes.

The goal of treatment is to lower the amount of protein leaking into your urine. In addition to lowering your blood glucose levels, you may be told to lower your blood pressure by eating a low-salt diet or taking an ACE inhibitor or ARB (angiotensin II receptor blocker). These prescription medications lower blood pressure by blocking the hormones that constrict blood vessels. You may also have to avoid certain medications, such as ibuprofen, and anti-inflammatory drugs that may compromise kidney function. Getting a handle on microalbuminuria now is critical to avoiding kidney disease later on. If you don't, you may move on to other stages of kidney disease.

Proteinuria

If microalbuminuria is not controlled, the amount of protein in your urine will increase, and you will develop proteinuria, also known as macroalbuminuria or nephrotic syndrome. Your urine may appear foamy in the toilet, and you may experience swelling in your hands, feet, abdomen, or face. You may also feel tired and out of breath. But in some cases, you may have no symptoms. Only by doing a urine test at your doctor's office will you know for sure.

At this point, it will be harder to stave off the progression of kidney disease. But you can still prevent the symptoms from getting worse by controlling blood glucose and lowering blood pressure. Blood pressure should be below 130/80 mmHg, which is lower than that recommended for non-diabetics. Also, lowering your salt intake, losing weight, and getting some regular exercise can help slow the progression.

Kidney Failure

When your kidneys can no longer filter toxins from the blood and keep protein in it, you have developed kidney failure. You may have less appetite, have difficulty concentrating, and experience bouts of nausea and itchiness. As kidney function deteriorates further, you may notice that you lose weight easily. You may also experience vomiting, lethargy, and weakness in your legs. If you take insulin, you may notice that you need less because smaller amounts are being excreted.

Although you will be advised to still keep your blood pressure low, your doctor may suggest you reexamine your blood glucose goals. Trying to keep blood glucose levels as close to normal as possible puts you at greater risk for hypoglycemia and will no longer provide any protective benefits to your kidneys. You may also be put on a low-protein diet to help slow the loss of kidney function. Your doctor may also need to evaluate your potassium and salt levels to ensure you have proper balance of metabolites. It may also be wise to start considering your options in the event of end-stage renal disease.

End-Stage Renal Disease

When the damage to your kidneys becomes very severe, they will no longer function at all. You may experience swelling in the ankles and face, and you may feel tired from the accumulation of fluid around the heart and lungs. You may also have muscle cramps in your gastrointestinal tract, and muscle and fat can start wasting away. In addition, you may have confusion and lapses in memory.

Without proper kidney function, you need to find an alternative method for eliminating bodily wastes. You can choose from three options: hemodialysis, peritoneal dialysis, or a kidney transplant.

In dialysis, the blood is cleansed of impurities, without removing the blood cells you need. Most patients have hemodialysis, which involves hooking you up to a machine at a clinic that acts like an artificial kidney. The blood is removed from an artery, usually in the arm, and circulated through the machine, then returned to the body through a vein. The procedure is done three times a week for four to six hours at a time. Another option is peritoneal dialysis, in which a solution called dialysate is inserted into your abdominal cavity to collect waste. After a certain interval, the solution is drained, then repeated again every four to six hours.

A kidney transplant is usually the more effective treatment. During surgery, your failed kidney is removed and replaced with a healthy one from a living donor, or someone who has recently died. More than 90 percent of people who get a kidney transplant survive the first year. Twenty percent live more than ten years. But finding a donor can take time, and you do face the risk of your immune system rejecting the new kidney.

A Final Note on Nephropathy
Kidney disease is not an inevitable consequence of having diabetes. Routine checks of protein levels in your urine can help you keep tabs on the functioning of your kidney. Preventive measures like getting your blood glucose to a normal range, keeping your blood pressure at healthy levels, and following a healthy diet that keeps your weight down can also help you avoid kidney failure.

Infections

In healthy people, the immune system is constantly on the lookout for invading microorganisms that could potentially harm your body. Once spotted, these germs are quickly eliminated. If they aren't destroyed, you develop an infection.

In people who have diabetes, the function of the immune system is weakened for reasons that remain unclear. The white blood cells that attack germs are less effective and the excess glucose provides a food supply for invading microorganisms. Other complications of diabetes can make you more susceptible to infections, too. Impaired blood flow can slow down the movement of white blood cells to the site of an impending infection. You'll be less likely to sense the discomfort caused by an infection if you have neuropathy. If you can't feel an injury to your foot, the wound is more likely to become infected.

A simple infection has several ramifications for a person with diabetes, not the least of which is hyperglycemia. If you have an infection, your body goes into overdrive to get rid of it, which can cause blood glucose levels to increase. Infections also give rise to stress, which in turn triggers the release of glucose from the liver and stimulates insulin resistance.

The infections can crop up anywhere in the body. The following areas may be especially vulnerable:

- *Gums and mouth.* Diabetics are more prone to peridontal disease than the general population. The disease arises from the bacteria growing between your gums and teeth, and can cause teeth and gums to separate. Eventually, teeth can become dislodged. The discomfort caused by gum disease can pose additional challenges for managing blood glucose if it interferes with regular eating patterns.
- *Ears.* Men who have diabetes may develop malignant external otitis, a bacterial infection of the ear. Although serious, the

condition does not indicate cancer, and is more common in men over age 65 who have had diabetes for a long time.

- *Urinary tract.* When the urinary tract is loaded up with glucose, microorganisms that thrive on sugar are apt to proliferate. The risk is higher if you're a woman, elderly, or have had diabetes for a long time. It's also higher if you have a neurogenic bladder that you have a hard time emptying, and in which the bacteria in the urine is allowed to linger.
- *Vaginal infections.* Some women who have diabetes are more prone to vaginal yeast infections. Candida albicans, the most common type of yeast infection, thrives in a moist environment nourished by large amounts of glucose.

Complications of the Feet

Your feet deserve some extra attention and tender loving care, especially if you have diabetes. In people with the disease, the feet are prime spots for complications. Bad circulation caused by problems in the blood vessels can restrict blood flow to the feet. Neuropathy may interfere with normal sensations, making it difficult for you to sense pain, calluses, ulcers, or corns. Without enough circulation and a reduction in sensation, these problems may be slow to heal, and your feet may be at risk for infections. Untreated infections can cause deformities, or even the loss of a limb.

Preventing Foot Problems

Diabetics can prevent foot problems by keeping blood glucose levels in a normal range, lowering high blood pressure, and having a doctor check their feet regularly. But having the disease means you should pay special attention to your feet by checking your feet daily, wearing well-fitted shoes, and immediately treating any problems that arise. Even a tiny sore can erupt into a serious infection if it goes untreated. Here's what the American Diabetes Association suggests you do to care for your feet:

- *Always keep your feet clean and dry.* Wash them every day with a mild soap, and dry carefully, especially between the toes.
- *If the skin on your feet is dry, apply a thin layer of lotion,* making sure to avoid the space between toes.
- *Put on fresh, clean socks or stockings every day.*
- *Inspect your feet and between toes daily for swelling, redness, cuts, or breaks.* Check your feet for extreme temperature differences. Extremely cold regions could indicate bad circulation, while very warm regions could suggest an infection.
- *Never go barefoot.* If you step on an object, and you have reduced feeling in your feet, you may not notice.
- *Cut your toenails straight across to avoid ingrown nails.*
- *Always wear comfortable shoes.* When trying on shoes, make sure they're comfortable immediately. Don't expect to break in a new pair of shoes. Leather shoes are generally better for your circulation.
- *If you do have neuropathy in your feet, don't trust yourself to know whether a shoe fits.* Find a shoe specialist who is trained to fit people with diabetes.
- *Always get early treatment for foot problems.* Call your doctor immediately if you see an open sore (ulcer); infection in a cut or blister; a red, tender toe; a change in feeling, such as pain, tingling, numbness, or burning; or a puncture wound caused by a nail or thorn.

Keeping Complications at Bay

Frightening as they may be, most complications from diabetes can be avoided or at least minimized with proper care, mainly by living a healthy lifestyle. As the Diabetes Control and Complications Trial showed, patients who monitor their blood glucose closely and try to keep it as close to normal as possible are better able to prevent or delay complications such as retinopathy, nerve damage, and cardiovascular disease. More specifically, the patients who practiced intensive management reduced the risk for retinopathy by 76 percent, kidney disease by 50 percent, and neuropathy by 60 percent.

The key points to remember are:

- Try to get your blood glucose as close to normal as possible.
- Lower high blood pressure, if you have it.
- Adopt strategies to lower your cholesterol, such as eating less saturated fat and more high-fiber foods.
- Do whatever you can to quit smoking.
- Incorporate some regular physical activity into your schedule.
- Lose weight, if you're too heavy.

Remember, these strategies will not only help you prevent or delay complications of diabetes. They'll also help improve your overall quality of life.

PERSONAL STORIES

Richard

Dismissing a diagnosis of diabetes is never a good idea. For Richard, a fifty-eight-year-old writer, ignoring the diagnosis for eight years finally landed him on the operating table where surgeons tried to revive the circulation in his legs and feet with bypass surgery.

Richard first learned he had diabetes in 1995. He had just broken his ankle and went in for surgery when blood tests revealed he had high blood sugar. The operation was temporarily postponed until his blood sugar was eventually lowered.

"The problem with diabetes is, you have no idea you have it," Richard says. "And I had no idea I had it."

Doctors gave him a prescription for insulin and taught him how to inject it. But at the time, Richard was trapped in a state of depression. Doctors warned him of the possibility of a silent heart attack from the diabetes, but Richard didn't care. Richard used the insulin for only a couple weeks then stopped, choosing to take his chances at the risk of losing his life.

A few years later, he had an attack of gout, a type of arthritis. He went to the hospital to get medication and was told once again that he had diabetes. Again, after two weeks on insulin, Richard chose to ignore his condition.

Finally, in the spring of 2003, Richard awoke one morning to find his feet tingling, feeling as if they'd fallen asleep. "It didn't go away the whole day," he says. "And over the next month or so, I would get sharp pains in my calves while I was walking. I had been okay about dying, but I would have liked to walk."

A vascular surgeon checked the circulation in his feet and found that there was none. Richard was diagnosed with neuropathy and ordered to undergo an operation the next day that would restore circulation to his right leg.

This time, when he saw how worried his wife was, Richard finally got serious about his health. The doctor gave him a prescription for Avandia and told him to come in for monthly checks of his blood glucose. He was also prescribed Lipitor to lower his high cholesterol.

He is now working on eating better by reducing his caloric intake to about 2,000 calories a day, avoiding the rich desserts that used to be a part of his nightly dinner, and eating more vegetables. And even while he is recovering from surgery, he has started exercising, something he once hated.

For Richard, the long delay in taking care of himself led to a serious complication, one that he must live with for the rest of his life. "I was told that the pains in my calf will go away, but the neuropathy in my feet will never go away," he says.

Though he isn't one to live with regrets, he knows that the way he chooses to live can take a toll on those who love him. "I didn't want to become a patient, but it just seems to be the price of making my wife feel better," he says. "And I don't want to be a burden to others."

Mike

Twenty-five years after he was diagnosed with diabetes, Mike developed retinopathy.

It had never been easy for Mike to control his blood glucose levels. For most of his adults years, he was overweight by as much as forty pounds, though that fluctuated depending on the time of year. He also had high cholesterol and high blood pressure.

"I was never really great about taking care of myself," says Mike, who works in advertising. "I knew that it was important to keep my blood sugars in a healthy range, but I just couldn't seem to do it right. I loved eating sweets and fried foods, and I really didn't enjoy vegetables. And I didn't have the time to exercise. So I let things go, and now I have to pay the price."

It wasn't as if Mike didn't try. When he was first diagnosed at the age of forty, he went on a diet and quickly shed fifteen pounds. He also started exercising by walking and biking. But as the years went on, and his career got busy, it became more difficult to remain disciplined. He and his wife divorced, and Mike sank into a deep depression. On top of feeling sad about losing his wife, he became terribly depressed about having diabetes. The bad feelings prompted him to eat more, and the weight came back.

"I hated going to the doctor all the time," he says. "And he put me on medication, too, which I didn't like taking. It just seemed so unfair that so many bad things were happening to me."

His doctor finally suggested he see a psychiatrist about his depression. The psychiatrist put him on an antidepressant, which worked wonders to alleviate the depression. Mike also met a new woman, another diabetic, who helped him feel better about himself. His new girlfriend served as a good role model because, unlike him, she was careful and had her blood glucose under control.

But for Mike, years of neglect had started to take its toll. Mike was now starting to notice blurry vision, which he simply attributed to age. When his new girlfriend suggested he see an ophthalmologist to make sure it wasn't something else, Mike took her advice and went. It had been years since he saw an eye doctor, and sure enough, the ophthalmologist detected retinopathy.

Fortunately for Mike, the disease was in its early stages and still nonproliferative. A single session of laser therapy helped heal most of the blood vessels, and Mike's vision improved. He is now more vigilant about taking care of his health. His doctor has put him on insulin to make sure he gets control of his blood glucose, and he's also started making some lifestyle changes. He gave up eating dessert and fried foods and makes sure to eat a lot of fruits and vegetables every day. He also takes a nightly walk with his girlfriend.

"I don't think I really believed it before when people said you had to watch your blood glucose or you'd have complications down the road," Mike says. "I always thought, 'It won't happen to me.' But look how wrong I was. Ultimately, I think I got lucky because it was still treatable when I caught it."

CHAPTER TEN

Gestational Diabetes

You've sweated through the nausea of the first trimester, felt the first kicks of your growing baby, and maybe even discovered whether you're having a boy or girl. Then, sometime in the sixth month, you get the stunning news: You have gestational diabetes.

Now what, you might be wondering. You didn't have diabetes before you got pregnant. How did this happen? How will this affect my baby's health? What about my health? What will this mean after my pregnancy?

Gestational diabetes afflicts about 2 percent of all pregnant women, or approximately 135,000 a year. The increased energy demands of a growing fetus causes the mother's body to produce large amounts of hormones to help the baby grow. Among them is a hormone called placental lactogen, a hormone produced by the placenta that, along with a genetic predisposition, is believed to play a role in causing gestational diabetes. These hormones block the effectiveness of insulin, causing the mom to become insulin-resistant and glucose to build up in the bloodstream.

In healthy pregnant women, the body manufactures enough insulin to overcome this resistance. The extra insulin helps move the glucose out of the blood and provides the energy your body needs in pregnancy. In women who develop gestational diabetes, the body can't produce enough to make up for the resistance.

Certain women are more likely to develop gestational diabetes than others. Women who are twenty-five years old or older, overweight at conception, and have a family history of diabetes are at greater risk for gestational diabetes. The condition is also more common among women who are Hispanic, Native American, African American, Asian American, or a Pacific Islander. In addition, you're at greater risk if you've already given birth to a stillborn or a baby weighing nine pounds or more, or were yourself a large baby at birth.

Fortunately, most women who have gestational diabetes go on to deliver healthy babies and experience no complications from this condition. The condition also usually disappears after birth, though the risk of developing Type 2 diabetes rises. But if it isn't closely monitored, and your blood sugars become too high, it can pose dangers to your unborn baby, and raise the odds you will deliver by caesarean section.

How Do I Know I Have It?

Chances are, you won't. That's because the symptoms of gestational diabetes resemble those of pregnancy. The frequent need to urinate, excessive thirst, and fatigue are all symptoms in pregnancy that are easily overlooked.

For that reason, obstetrician/gynecologists usually test for gestational diabetes sometime between the twenty-fourth and twenty-eighth week of pregnancy using the oral glucose tolerance test. That's when hormones from the placenta start to interfere with the function of insulin. For the test, you will be asked to drink a sweet, syrupy beverage loaded with fifty grams of glucose, at least double the amount of sugar in a soda the same size. Blood is then drawn and analyzed. If blood sugar levels are higher than normal, gestational diabetes is suspected, and further tests are done.

The second test is considerably more elaborate. In the three days before the test, the woman is required to eat 150 grams of carbohydrates a day, the equivalent of about one cup of pasta, two or three servings of fruit, four slices of bread, and three glasses of milk. Ten to fourteen hours before the test, you cannot eat or drink anything except water. A blood sample is then taken to measure fasting blood glucose levels. The patient then drinks a solution with 100 grams of glucose. Blood samples are drawn every hour for three hours. If two samples contain higher than normal blood sugar levels, the patient is said to have gestational diabetes.

Treating Gestational Diabetes

Like all forms of diabetes, treating gestational diabetes involves trying to get blood glucose levels as close to normal as possible. A woman with gestational diabetes should aim to get her blood sugars down to the same level as a pregnant woman without the condition.

Most women can control their diabetes through diet and exercise. But if blood glucose levels do not drop, your doctor may also prescribe insulin to compensate for the insulin your body is unable to produce. Insulin does not cross the placenta. Because drugs can cross the placenta and get into the baby's blood, pregnant women are not prescribed oral medications.

One of the most important aspects of your treatment will be close monitoring of your blood glucose. Your doctor may ask you to use home test kits that let you do self-monitoring in addition to more frequent visits to the physician's office for blood glucose checks.

Diet and Exercise

If you have been diagnosed with gestational diabetes, you should work out a meal plan with a registered dietitian that will help lower blood glucose levels. You may need to learn to eat different foods, practice better portion control and strategies to limit weight gain during the rest of your pregnancy. You should strive for a well-balanced diet that includes plenty of fruits, vegetables, and grains, but limited servings of high-fat, high-sugar foods.

Women with gestational diabetes should also try to incorporate some form of exercise into their routine. Exercise helps lower blood glucose levels by making body cells more sensitive to the effects of insulin. Be sure to follow these precautions to ensure a safe workout:

- Consult your doctor before starting an exercise regimen. Ask for ideas on how to do low-intensity exercises that are safe and beneficial. Some possible exercises might include swimming, water aerobics, and stationary bicycling.
- If you weren't exercising before your pregnancy, don't start doing strenuous workouts now.
- Drink plenty of fluids before, during, and after you exercise.
- Warm up before and cool down after a workout.
- Limit the most strenuous part of your exercise to just fifteen minutes.
- Keep your heart rate below 140 beats per minute while you exercise.
- Avoid exercises that involve lying on your back, straining or holding your breath, or jerky movements and quick changes in direction.
- If you feel lightheaded, weak, or out of breath, stop exercising immediately.
- Learn to feel for uterine contractions during exercise. These contractions are an indication that you may be overdoing it.

Getting Additional Medical Help

If you are diagnosed with gestational diabetes, your ob/gyn might recommend you find some other health professionals to help manage your care. In addition to a registered dietitian, you might want to consult with a certified diabetes educator to learn how to monitor your blood glucose. You may also want to talk to an exercise physiologist about devising a safe exercise regimen. In addition, you may need to enlist a neonatologist to help you address any complications that might occur with your baby at birth.

Possible Complications from Gestational Diabetes

Having gestational diabetes does put you at risk for certain complications. But fortunately, these complications are preventable and manageable. Good blood glucose control, a healthy diet, and reasonable weight gain can all help improve your odds of having a healthy delivery and baby. Still, you should know what the complications are.

Macrosomia

During pregnancy, the fetus relies on the mother for all its nutrients, and gets it from the mother's blood. If that blood contains excess glucose, the fetus's pancreas goes into overdrive to produce insulin to use up that glucose. So while the mother may not be able to make enough insulin, the fetus can.

But rather than burn it up for energy, the glucose is converted into fat, which causes your baby to grow larger and fatter in the womb. The result is macrosomia, which literally means large body. A baby with macrosomia is at greater risk for delivery by caesarean section. In some cases, the baby needs to be delivered early. Large babies delivered early are at greater risk for having health problems such as respiratory distress because the lungs are not mature yet.

Preeclampsia

Women with gestational diabetes are at greater risk for developing preeclampsia, also called toxemia, a condition in which blood pressure gets too high. As a result, you may experience swelling in your feet and lower legs, and leaking of protein into your urine. You may notice sudden weight gain and develop headaches, nausea, vomiting, abdominal pain, and blurry vision. Preeclampsia is usually detected by a blood pressure check or with a urine test.

If you are diagnosed with preeclampsia, you may be confined to bed rest for the duration of your pregnancy, but the only real cure is delivery of the baby. Your doctor will regularly monitor your blood pressure, and you may be asked to take your own blood pressure at home. Your ob/gyn may also examine you and the baby to determine whether a premature delivery is viable. The condition is very serious and if untreated, can cause seizures, coma, and death to you or your baby.

Hypoglycemia

A baby born to a mother with gestational diabetes is at risk for experiencing hypoglycemia immediately after delivery. If the mother's blood sugar has been consistently high during the pregnancy, the baby will have high levels of insulin in circulation. After delivery, the high insulin levels persist, but the baby no longer has the high level of sugar coming from its mother. As a result, the newborn's blood sugar will fall to lower levels. If the baby's blood glucose levels continue to be low after birth, intravenous doses of glucose may be necessary.

Jaundice

Another risk for babies is jaundice, a condition that can also occur in babies born to women without gestational diabetes. During gestation, your baby produces large amounts of red blood cells that are no longer needed after delivery. The red blood cells are then broken down, a process that produces bilirubin. The bilirubin is then processed by the liver and eliminated.

If the baby's liver isn't mature enough, the process cannot be accomplished, and the bilirubin lingers in the baby's body, producing a yellowish hue in the baby's skin. The yellow coloring is called jaundice. The condition is usually treated in the hospital by placing the baby under special lights that eliminate the bilirubin.

High Ketones

If you have gestational diabetes, you should check your urine for ketones, toxic acids produced by the body from the breakdown of fats for energy. High levels of ketones are more likely to develop if you aren't drinking enough fluids or eating enough food to satisfy your extra energy demands. Both you and the baby are at greater risk then for ketoacidosis, which can lead to seizures, coma, and death.

Urinary Tract Infection

High levels of blood glucose can make you prone to urinary tract infections, which are usually caused by bacteria. These bacteria thrive in the sugar-rich environment caused by high blood glucose. You may notice that you need to urinate more frequently, or that urine is cloudy or bloody. You may also experience, fever, abdominal pain, and chills.

What the Future Holds

Fortunately, gestational diabetes usually goes away after the baby is born, and the placenta is delivered. Your physician will test your blood glucose levels to make sure. Some health-care providers will do an oral glucose tolerance test six to eight weeks after delivery to check for diabetes.

But your risk for having diabetes in the future does go up. For instance, in subsequent pregnancies, you have a 70 percent chance of having gestational diabetes again. You also have a 40 to 60 percent chance of developing Type 2 diabetes in five to fifteen years. And if you're obese, your odds of having Type 2 diabetes in the future rises to 75 percent.

What Can I Do?

Just because you had gestational diabetes doesn't mean you are helpless to avoid diabetes later on. But it does increase your risk. You can take steps to reduce the risk in your favor by following these basic rules:

- *Lose weight.* Getting your weight to a healthy range will lower the odds you'll have diabetes.
- *Eat a healthy, well-balanced diet.* Restrict your intake of unhealthy foods, while trying to eat more fruits, vegetables, and grains.
- *Exercise.* Physical activity makes your body more sensitive to the effects of insulin and lowers glucose levels. It also helps promote weight loss.

PERSONAL STORIES

Alexis: In Her Own Words

When I first started developing symptoms of diabetes, all I remember is being thirsty all the time, even after just having a couple glasses of water. My throat felt like a desert. No matter how much I drank, I was never satisfied.

For several months I also noticed an increased need to urinate. I had no energy and was losing weight for no apparent reason. My grandfather was a Type 1 diabetic, so I knew that diabetes ran in the family. One day in seventh grade health class I skipped ahead to the chapter that talked about diabetes. After only a few paragraphs, I was convinced I knew why I hadn't been feeling well. I confronted my mother with my fears, but she completely disregarded them. "Don't be silly," she told me. "When I was young, your grandmother was always dragging me off for glucose tolerance tests and there was never anything wrong with me. Believe me, if you had diabetes, you'd be a lot sicker."

As a child I had always been prone to melodrama—they used to call me Sarah Bernhardt—and my mom attributed my fears to more of these histrionics. So I didn't completely blame my mom for thinking I'd gone overboard with my self-diagnosis. In response, I told her I'd just wait it out and then they'd see there was something really wrong with me. She thought it was just more high drama. Looking back, I wonder if she was afraid of discovering the truth.

It was on a weekend class trip to the Ashland, Oregon, Shakespeare Festival that my mom grew truly worried about my health. What was supposed to be a four-hour drive turned into a six-hour journey, with all the extra pit stops I had to make. By this point, I was drinking nearly two gallons of water a day and urinating up to twenty-five times in a twenty-four-hour period. At the hotel where my mom and I shared a room, she was awakened several times as I got up every hour to use the bathroom. She quickly realized that this behavior wasn't normal. When I finally had a glucose test, the results were extremely high. My family made an appointment with a doctor, and within a few days I was in the hospital, a newly diagnosed diabetic.

Right from the start, my doctors discussed my fertility. It was the early 1990s when I was diagnosed, and most experts still believed that diabetics should avoid pregnancy. As a thirteen-year-old girl, getting pregnant was not exactly on my mind, but the nurses and doctors thought it best to warn me in advance. They probably thought it was better to crush any hope in me right away, rather than have me hold out hope that would never manifest. "You'll never have children," they told me. "Besides, you'll probably never marry, seeing that no man in his right mind would marry an infertile woman."

Looking back, their remarks sound as if they came from the dark ages—not a mere fifteen years ago. But ignorance about diabetes and pregnancy still persists. Remember the movie *Steel Magnolias*? A diabetic woman (played by Julia Roberts), against the advice of her doctor and family, gets pregnant, has a healthy baby, and then dies of complications from diabetes. Fifty years ago that may have been true. Thankfully, things have changed.

Just a few years ago at one of my regular appointments with my diabetes specialist at the Joslin Clinic in Boston, I was told, "We have a fantastic pregnancy clinic here. Whenever you're ready, ask us to set up an appointment for you." I couldn't believe my ears. Me? Have a baby? But I'm diabetic, I thought. He replied as if he'd read my mind: "No problem, just make sure to have an appointment before you get pregnant." "But I was told that I could never have children," I said, still puzzled. "Nonsense," he insisted, "Times have changed. There's absolutely no reason why you shouldn't bask in the glow of motherhood as other women do." His remarks changed everything for me. That afternoon, I had visions of grandchildren happily playing in my mother's lap.

What I have learned over the years is that with good glucose control, a woman with diabetes can have a safe, healthy pregnancy and birth. In fact, proper long-term care can help you dodge most complications of diabetes. It isn't easy, I know. Even something so simple as going to the gym can force me to think about how I'm controlling my blood sugars. Because I'm prone to high blood glucose after exercise, I usually need an insulin injection before working out.

I don't know about you, but I plan to be having a fabulous time in my old age: searching piles of junk at Eastern European flea markets for hidden treasures, hiking the Appalachians, dancing at my youngest brother's wedding. Whatever your pearl may be, the instructions are clear—take care of your diabetes by controlling your blood glucose, and the world is truly your oyster.

—*Alexis M.*

Jane

At forty-five, Jane looks like a pillar of good health. She exercises almost every day. She follows a well-balanced diet, with only an occasional sweet. She also does meditation twice a week to help keep stress levels in check.

But her healthy lifestyle was not always the way she lived. In her twenties, Jane was overweight, carrying nearly 200 pounds on her 5-foot, 3-inch frame. With a busy career as public relations executive, she was always eating on the run, opting for fast foods that were high in fat and calories. She got little exercise and barely had time to sleep. She was always under a lot of stress.

When she got pregnant at age thirty-one, Jane got the wake-up call she needed. "I found out I had gestational diabetes," Jane says. "I felt terrible, and I was terrified for my unborn baby. That's when I became super conscientious about everything I ate and did."

During her pregnancy, Jane kept close watch over blood glucose levels and began eating more carefully. She started by cutting back on the fast foods and desserts. She also stopped eating late at night. And though she hadn't done much exercise before, Jane started taking short little walks, ten minutes at a time, just to get in the habit of exercising.

Despite her vigilance, Jane gave birth to a relatively large baby boy who weighed nine pounds, twelve ounces. She did it by C-section. "I was so relieved when he arrived," she says. "The diabetes had scared me so much because now I knew it could affect someone else."

Even after the pregnancy, the prospect of having diabetes haunted her. "I kept asking myself, 'Why hadn't I done a better job of taking care of myself before I got pregnant?'" Jane says. "Why was I so caught up in everything else in my life that I wasn't taking care of my health? The worst part is, I have a family history of diabetes. My grandfather had it, and so did my aunt. I should have been much more careful."

Jane vowed that she was going to take better care of herself, especially since she knew that there was a likelihood she'd have diabetes someday. She started going to Weight Watchers and learning how to eat better. She gave up refined sugars, soda, and high-fat munchies that used to keep her company while she watched TV. She also started exercising at a gym and working with a personal trainer who taught her how to use weights.

The pounds began coming off, and a year later, Jane was down to 140 pounds. She felt better than ever and decided to get pregnant again. Because she'd had gestational diabetes with her first pregnancy, the doctors started testing her blood glucose early on.

Her hard work paid off: Jane never got gestational diabetes the second time. She gave birth to a healthy eight-pound girl. "I couldn't believe it," she says. "I thought for sure I was doomed, given my family history. But I learned that taking care of myself can make all the difference in the world."

Today, Jane continues to abide by her diet and exercise routines. Though she no longer has to lose a lot of weight and is strictly in maintenance mode, she still watches what she eats. She has also become an avid walker and gardener, and still does weight-training three times a week. Best of all, she's been able to steer clear of diabetes.

CHAPTER ELEVEN

Sexual Health and Diabetes

Learning you have diabetes may not put you in the mood for romance with your favorite squeeze. It may also make you think twice about having children. Or you may find it wreaks havoc on your monthly bouts with PMS. Unfortunately, diabetes can present physical complications that will affect your sexual health and well-being.

More specifically, too much glucose in your blood can cause erectile dysfunction (ED) in men, make women more susceptible to vaginal dryness, and put a major damper on your libido or sexual interest. To make matters worse, you may be uncomfortable even calling attention to these problems with your doctor. But only by discussing these concerns with your physician will you be able to improve your sexual well-being. That's why an entire chapter is devoted to your sexual health and diabetes.

Blood Glucose and Menstruation

It's bad enough that you must endure the mood swings every month. The cravings for unhealthy foods. The uncomfortable bloating and annoying cramps. As a diabetic, you may now also be prone to fluctuations in your blood glucose levels as well.

For reasons that remain unclear, a woman's monthly menstrual cycle affects her ability to control blood glucose. If it's any comfort, the problem is not uncommon. According to one survey of 200 women with Type 1 diabetes, 27 percent had problems with high blood glucose in the week before their periods. Another 12 percent had trouble with low blood glucose in that same time. In a separate survey of 700 women, 70 percent said they experienced problems with blood glucose control in the premenstrual period. Of course, the surveys do not account for diet and exercise, but they do suggest that there's a connection between your monthly cycle and having the disease.

Menstruation and Diabetes

Every month, from the time she reaches menarche in early adolescence until she reaches menopause in her late forties or early fifties, a woman's body undergoes the amazing process of preparing itself to reproduce and achieve pregnancy. The process is known as the menstrual cycle, and it involves four distinct events:

- *Menstruation.* Also known as your monthly period, menstruation occurs when the uterine lining is shed, along with blood and secretions from the vagina and cervix. The uterine lining thickens every month in anticipation of pregnancy. But if an egg is not fertilized, the lining is shed, and menstruation begins.
- *Follicular phase.* Menstruation occurs during the follicular phase. On the day your period starts, the follicle-stimulating hormone goes into production, which in turn stimulates the production of estrogen. Approximately twelve to fourteen days later, the effects of estrogen kick into full gear, causing an ovary to release an egg.
- *Ovulation.* Once the egg is released, it travels down the fallopian tube and begins its journey toward the uterus, a process that takes about six days. While in transit, the egg is subject to

fertilization by sperm. Fertilization can take place within twenty-four hours after ovulation.

- *Luteal phase.* This phase begins at ovulation and ends with menstruation. Once the egg is released, a second hormone called luteinizing hormone triggers the ovary to produce estrogen and progesterone. The hormones trigger the uterine lining to thicken and to start storing nutrients in the event there's a fertilized egg. If an egg is fertilized, pregnancy occurs. But if it goes unfertilized, the lining is shed, and menstruation begins.

The Impact of Diabetes

During the luteal phase, as estrogen and progesterone surges through your body, you may experience difficulties managing your blood glucose. You may notice this difficulty at the same time other symptoms of premenstrual syndrome or PMS appear. In some women, the high blood glucose occurs in the morning, and is then followed by low blood glucose in the mid-morning.

No one knows exactly why this occurs, but one theory is that the hormones affect the way a woman's body deals with insulin. The increase in hormones appears to make body cells more resistant to the effects of insulin. If cells are more resistant, then you are more likely to have higher levels of blood glucose.

Not everyone believes hormones are at the root of this increase in blood glucose. Some experts link the rise to the symptoms of PMS, which include irritability, bloating, and cravings for fats and carbohydrates.

In some women, the hormones have the opposite effect, and body cells are actually more sensitive to insulin. As a result, blood glucose levels may actually fall in the week before menstruation. In any case, many women appear to experience changes in blood glucose levels in the week before their periods.

How Do I Know It's My Period?

Close monitoring of blood glucose and good record keeping can help you determine whether your monthly period is wreaking havoc on your diabetes. Jot down your blood glucose levels, and mark the date your period begins. If you've been keeping a log book with your blood glucose readings, try to go back and write down those dates. Also make notes of any symptoms of PMS, such as bloating, irritability, weight gain, fatigue, cramps, and food cravings.

Continue keeping your records for several months, then go back and review the information. Look for patterns in your blood glucose readings. Are they higher than usual in the week before your period? Do they drop? Or are they relatively stable the entire month? Do they change at the same time you develop symptoms of PMS?

Reducing the PMS Factor

One way to help reduce the impact of your monthly cycle on blood glucose levels is to get a handle on PMS. This may help you avoid the cravings for high-fat, high-carbohydrate foods that can also send blood glucose upward. Here are some strategies:

- *Watch your diet.* Limit your intake of salt, which can cause fluid retention. And follow your diabetic meal plan closely, so you can keep blood glucose as close to normal as possible.
- *Eat at consistent times every day.* Skipping meals and erratic snacking can cause blood glucose levels to swing. These erratic shifts in blood glucose can exacerbate some of the symptoms of PMS, which in turn can worsen blood glucose control.
- *Avoid too much chocolate, caffeine, and alcohol in your diet.* These foods are stimulants that can affect your blood glucose. They can also affect your emotional well-being, making you prone to the symptoms of PMS.
- *Get regular exercise.* Physical activity helps reduce the impact of PMS and regulate blood glucose levels.

If blood glucose levels continue to remain high in the days before your period, consider doing some extra exercise, eating fewer carbohydrates, and perhaps increasing your dosage of insulin.

If Blood Glucose Rises
Some women experience a rise in blood glucose around the time they get their periods. You can counter this increase by getting more exercise, eating less carbohydrates, or increasing your insulin dosage. If you want to adjust your insulin, you should consult your doctor first. The increase in dosage is usually small and should correspond with the rise in blood glucose near the end of your cycle.

If Blood Glucose Falls
In some women, their monthly periods can coincide with dips in blood glucose. Adjusting insulin or diabetes medications in the days before they get their periods can sometimes help, but you should always talk to your doctor first before making these changes. You may also cut back on your exercise in that time or increase your intake of carbohydrates.

The Irregular Cycle
Not all women are blessed with a predictable menstrual cycle. For some women, their periods are erratic and unpredictable, making it hard for them to determine when they'll even get their periods until a telltale signal like breast tenderness provides a clue. In others, there may be no such clue, and it becomes hard to know whether monthly menstrual cycles are affecting blood glucose levels.

The only way to know is to figure out when you are ovulating. There are several ways to determine when you ovulate. They are:

- *Check for vaginal secretions.* Shortly after your period, you typically have no vaginal secretions. But as you approach ovulation, you may notice a clear discharge. And when ovulation occurs, the discharge may become thicker and stickier.

188

- *Chart your basal body temperature.* Before ovulation, your body temperature usually falls 0.5 to 1.0 degrees. When you are actually ovulating, the temperature can rise 0.5 to 1.5 degrees. Mark the date your temperature rises. Since the time between ovulation and the onset of menstruation is usually fourteen days, you should be able to pinpoint the timing of your next period. You should take your temperature in the morning for about two minutes before you get out of bed.
- *Use an ovulation predictor kit.* Using a simple urine test, an ovulation predictor kit can tell you when you ovulate. The kits are costly but available over-the-counter in most drugstores.

Sex and Diabetes

Having diabetes is hardly the kind of thing that jumpstarts your libido. In fact, it can have just the opposite effect. You may feel anxious, depressed, and overwhelmed about having a chronic condition. The rigors of managing this disease can sabotage your sex drive. The medications you take to relieve pain or combat depression can also suppress your desire.

Physically, you may experience problems and complications that can impede sexual performance. If you have bad circulation or neuropathy caused by diabetes, you may not have enough blood flow to the vagina or penis. Without enough blood flow, women may experience pain and irritation during sex. If you're a man, you may have trouble with impotence.

One of the best things you can do for your sex life is to get your blood glucose under control. If your blood glucose is not well managed, you may feel too tired to have sex in the first place. It can also worsen some other sexual problems.

Sex and Hypoglycemia

If you do have sex, you might be at risk for hypoglycemia, especially if you use insulin. Like any physical activity, sex burns calories and requires energy. Overexertion can cause blood glucose to dip to low levels, putting you at risk for hypoglycemia. Here are some steps to take to prevent a bout of low blood sugars during sex:

- Take your blood glucose before having sex. It's not the most romantic thing in the world, but it can spare you the trouble later of dealing with low blood sugar. If your blood sugar is low or normal, and you tend to exert a lot of energy during sex, have a small snack beforehand.
- Eat a snack after sex to bring blood glucose back up.
- If you use an insulin pump, consider disconnecting it, so your blood sugar doesn't fall too low. If you're active during sex, the activity might be enough to control blood glucose. Talk to your doctor first, and find out how long you can keep it detached.

Physical Challenges of Sex for Women

Both men and women who have diabetes may experience certain physical difficulties when it comes to sex. Here's how a woman's sex life might be affected:

- *Loss of sensation.* When diabetes causes damage to the nerves, you may experience a loss of feeling in your sexual organs. The diminished sensation can cause low arousal and difficulties achieving orgasm. Changing the way your body is stimulated may help.
- *Vaginal dryness.* Nerve damage to the cells lining your vagina can also cause vaginal dryness, which can lead to irritation, pain, and discomfort during sex. In women who have reached menopause, the reduction in sex hormones can naturally bring on more dryness, which will only exacerbate the problem.
- *Vaginal infections.* Women who have diabetes are prone to developing yeast infections. The extra blood glucose is a breeding

ground for yeast to grow and thrive. Most of these infections are caused by candida albicans, a fungus. If you have vaginal infections, you may notice a discharge, itching, burning, redness and swelling in your vaginal area. Intercourse may be painful. Antifungal creams are generally used to treat vaginal infections. Oral medications like Diflucan 150 mg, which is just one pill, can also treat the infection.

- *Urinary tract infections.* Similarly, high blood glucose levels can cause infections in the urinary tract. Symptoms of a UTI include frequent urination, pain or burning during urination, cloudy or bloody urine, fever, and chills. Having sex while you have a urinary tract infection can be painful. UTIs are treated with antibiotics.

- *Loss of bladder control.* Nerve damage in the bladder can cause incontinence. You may not know when it's full and may experience leakage during intercourse. To prevent this, you should go to the bathroom before and after sex.

Men and Erectile Dysfunction

For men with diabetes, the biggest sexual problem is erectile dysfunction or impotence. Approximately 50 to 60 percent of diabetic men over the age of fifty will experience impotence. The problem is more prevalent among older men, but in men who have diabetes, impotence tends to occur ten to fifteen years earlier than it does in men without the disease.

Impotence is the inability to have or maintain an erection, making it impossible for you to have intercourse. Erectile dysfunction in diabetics is usually attributed to problems with the circulatory system or nervous system, so men who have had cardiovascular or neurological complications are at greater risk. Reduced blood flow to the penis can make it hard to stay erect. Problems in the nervous system can interfere with signals from the brain to the blood vessels that create an erection.

But impotence may also be the result of psychological issues, such as depression, anxiety, and stress. Too much stress can decrease your brain's response to testosterone, the male hormone that aids in achieving an erection. Even knowing that you might have a problem achieving an erection can make it difficult for you to do so.

In some cases, impotence can result from the use of certain medications, such as those used to treat high blood pressure, anxiety, depression, and peptic ulcers. Smoking cigarettes and drinking alcohol can also cause erectile dysfunction.

Treating Erectile Dysfunction

Before you can treat impotence, you need to find out if the cause is physical or psychological. One way to do that is to find out whether you are having erections in the middle of the night. Most healthy men have several erections while they are sleeping. By monitoring your erections in a sleep lab, you can find out if you're still capable of achieving a middle-of-the-night erection, which indicates you are physiologically fit. Testosterone levels should be checked and a thyroid test done before you assume it is depression or psychological. You can ask your doctor to perform these tests.

If you can't, then the problem may very well be physical, and you may need medical treatment. Several options exist:

- *Sildenafil (Viagra)*. Taken an hour before sexual intercourse, sildenafil works by relaxing the smooth muscle tissue in the penis, which increases blood flow and makes an erection easier to achieve. The drug continues to work for about four hours. But the drug does have side effects, including headache, facial flushing, and upset stomach. In higher doses, it can produce short-term visual problems, blurred vision, and light sensitivity. Sildenafil belongs to a class of medications known as PDE5 inhibitors, which now also includes vardenafil

(Levitra) and tadalafil (Cialis). These medications cannot be taken if you are already taking nitrates to lower your blood pressure. The combination can lower blood pressure to dangerous levels.

- *Alprostadil.* Alprostadil (also called MUSE, or medicated urethral system for erection) is a prostaglandin administered through the transurethral system as a urethral pellet. This medication mimics the actions of a naturally-occurring substance that is involved in the development of an erection. Alprostadil can be used with sildenafil if either one is not effective alone. The erection that results usually lasts thirty minutes to an hour. This medication may be placed into the urethra by inserting a suppository into the tip of the penis. Side effects include mild pain in some individuals. If you use an injection of alprostadil, you may develop a prolonged erection that is painful and can damage the tissue in your penis.

- *Vacuum devices.* If medications do not help, you may consider using a vacuum device. A plastic tube is placed over the penis, and using a hand pump, air is drawn out of the tube. In the process, blood is pulled into the penis, causing an erection. Once erect, you slip an elastic ring off the base of the tube and place it over your penis, trapping the blood inside. The device allows for a thirty-minute erection after which the ring should be immediately removed. Beyond that, sustained use of the ring can damage the tissue in the penis.

- *Surgical implants.* Another option is to surgically implant a penile prostheses that mimics the actions of a healthy penis during intercourse. Semi-rigid rod implants are permanently erect and must be adjusted depending on whether you're having intercourse or going about your day, while inflatable implants are erect only when inflated. Surgical implants have a risk for infection, and the devices are subject to breakage.

If the problem behind your erectile dysfunction is psychological, you should consult a therapist who specializes in issues of sexuality. Openly discussing the problem and pinpointing the root of your stress, depression, or anxiety may help alleviate impotence.

Birth Control

No one wants an unplanned pregnancy. But for women who have diabetes, the risk for birth defects increases substantially if blood glucose levels aren't well controlled before pregnancy. In fact, if you don't have blood glucose under control at the time you conceive, your odds of having a baby with birth defects increases from 2 percent to as high as 8 percent, which is a four-fold increase.

That's why birth control is so important to people who have the disease. Using the rhythm method, which relies on avoiding fertilization during ovulation, is not an option because it's not reliable enough. As a diabetic, you need something more dependable to make sure you do not become unexpectedly pregnant. There are several options.

Oral Contraception

In the years since they debuted in the U.S. in 1960, birth control pills have become the most popular method of contraception on the market. Their popularity is due in large part to their success rate. Used correctly, only 0.1 percent of women become pregnant. Taken as a whole and accounting for errors in usage, the pill has a success rate of 95 percent.

But women with diabetes have special concerns when it comes to oral contraception. Birth control pills contain hormones, which vary depending on the type of pill, and can affect your blood glucose levels.

- *Monophasic pills* contain fixed amounts of estrogen and progesterone that you take through your entire menstrual cycle.
- *Triphasic pills* contain doses of estrogen and progesterone that vary every seven days.

• *Progesterone-only contraceptives* contain only the one hormone and are taken every day. These medications are also available as injections, called Depo-Provera, which lasts for three months, and as implantable capsules called Norplant, which last for five years.

Which Pill Should I Use?

If you think you want to use an oral contraceptive, you should discuss that with your diabetes doctor as well as your OB/GYN. Progesterone-only contraceptives can raise blood glucose levels. You may want to use a short-term progesterone-only pill before trying one of the long-term forms of contraception. If you have Type 2 diabetes and are controlling it with diet alone, you may want to avoid this method of birth control because it could increase your need for insulin.

Monophasic and triphasic birth control pills appear to be safe for people with Type 1 or Type 2 diabetes who are keeping blood glucose at or near the normal range. But there are no studies demonstrating their long-term safety. These pills are riskier, however, if you are over thirty-five, smoke, and have a history of heart disease, stroke, high blood pressure, or peripheral blood vessel disease—all factors that elevate your risk for blood clot formation. You also raise your risk for retinopathy and kidney disease if you develop high blood pressure while using birth control pills. Injections and implants of progesterone-only contraceptives are usually safer in women who are older than thirty-five and have diabetes and/or vascular disease.

If you do opt to use birth control pills, monitor blood glucose closely, especially in the beginning. The pill may affect insulin sensitivity, and you may need to adjust your dosage accordingly. Also, be sure to have your doctor keep an eye on your blood pressure, cholesterol, and triglycerides. An increase in any of them may raise your risk for blood clots and prompt you to reconsider the use of the pill.

Intrauterine Device or IUD

An intrauterine device works by blocking an embryo, a fertilized egg, from implanting in the uterus. The T-shaped device is surgically inserted into the uterus and can remain in place for as long as nine years. Plastic IUDs release progesterone, and need to be replaced every year. The devices may increase your risk for vaginal infections and are generally not recommended for women with diabetes. Copper IUDs can remain in place for up to nine years and have not been associated with vaginal infections. IUDs are not recommended for women who have multiple sex partners or plan to have children in the future. In some women, IUDs may cause menstrual pain and irregularities.

Barrier Methods

The diaphragm, sponge, and cervical cap are barrier methods of contraception that prevent sperm from entering the uterus. The diaphragm is a rubber cap that is coated in spermicidal jelly, inserted into the vagina, and placed over the cervix. Its effectiveness depends largely on the user's ability to place it correctly. The sponge contains spermicidal jelly and is inserted into the vagina where like the diaphragm, it is placed over the cervix. The cervical cap is a small device that also fits over the cervix to block the entrance of sperm into the uterus.

Sterilization

If you're older or if you plan never to have children, sterilization may be an option. The procedure, also known as tubal ligation, divides the fallopian tubes, thereby preventing sperm from reaching the uterus. Done correctly, this method is 100 percent effective at preventing unwanted pregnancies.

Contraception for Men

The ability to prevent an unwanted pregnancy is not entirely a woman's job. Men have two options they can choose from.

Condoms

Condoms are rubber sheaths that are placed over an erect penis before intercourse. Upon ejaculation, the sperm is deposited in the tip of the rubber sheath and prevented from entering the uterus. Used correctly and with a spermicide, condoms are about 88 percent effective.

Vasectomy

Men who are finished having children or who do not intend to have them may consider a vasectomy. It takes less than one hour to do the procedure in the doctor's office or in an outpatient surgery center. The procedure prevents the release of sperm into the semen, so the semen that is ejaculated contains no sperm. But the man is still fully capable of ejaculating. Like sterilization in women, men should be certain that they do not want any more children because the procedure is difficult and expensive to reverse.

Pregnancy and Diabetes

Women who have diabetes have higher odds of a healthy pregnancy than they did in the past. Good preconception care, careful monitoring of blood glucose levels throughout pregnancy, and strategies to remain healthy all help lower the risk of birth defects, miscarriages, and still-births that used to haunt diabetic women who wanted to have children. The planning process begins before conception.

The Preconception Dos

You and your partner know you want to have children. Begin now, before you conceive, to take steps that will help you enjoy a safe and trouble-free pregnancy that results in a healthy baby:

- *Talk to your medical team.* Alert them to your plans, and discuss your concerns. Your doctor can help you identify challenges you might need to overcome before you get pregnant.

- *Get a thorough physical exam.* If your doctor finds out you have high blood pressure, or complications of the heart, eyes, kidney, or nerves, you may need to get treatment before conception. These complications can pose risks to the mother and the unborn baby.

   In some cases, such as kidney disease, retinopathy, or heart disease, you may be advised against getting pregnant. Kidney function can worsen in women with kidney disease who get pregnant, and preexisting heart problems can raise your risk for heart attack. If you have retinopathy, the condition may also worsen with pregnancy.
- *Have an HbA1C test done.* You need to know how well you are controlling your blood glucose levels over time. The closer it is to normal, the better your odds for a healthy pregnancy.
- *Get your blood glucose under control.* Poor glucose control can raise the risk for birth defects in your baby. Women with diabetes have a 6 to 12 percent chance of delivering a baby with birth defects, compared with healthy women who have a risk of 2 to 3 percent. Tight control of blood glucose before pregnancy, however, can lower that risk to as little as 1 percent, according to one study.

Reining in your blood glucose also helps you develop and practice the lifestyle strategies that you will need during your pregnancy. Healthy eating, regular exercise, and trying to keep weight gain in check will all be important to your well-being during pregnancy, as well as that of your unborn child. You should also have thyroid tests done before and during your pregnancy since hyperthyroidism and hypothyroidism are likely to occur.

In some cases, you may need insulin to help control blood glucose levels. If you are already using insulin, you may need to practice intensive management in order to get the levels under control.

Will My Baby Have Diabetes?

No doubt about it—one of your first concerns will be whether your child will inherit your condition. The odds vary a great deal, depending on which parent has diabetes, how long the parent has had it, the age of diagnosis, and the age of conception. More specifically, experts know:

- A baby born to a mother who has Type 1 diabetes and is over twenty-five years of age has a 1 percent chance of developing diabetes.
- If the mother is younger than twenty-five at the time of birth, the child's risk increases to 4 percent.
- If the father has Type 1 diabetes, the odds for the child go up to about 6 percent.
- The risk doubles if the parent with Type 1 diabetes was diagnosed before age eleven.
- If both parents have Type 1 diabetes, the risk is undetermined, but probably higher.
- The risk is less specific in Type 2 diabetes, but the disease is usually a combination of lifestyle factors and a genetic predisposition.
- Just because a child has a family history of Type 2 diabetes does not mean the child will have it, too. Lifestyle factors, such as healthy eating and regular physical activity, can usually compensate for genetic susceptibility.

During Pregnancy

Once you do become pregnant, you need to remain vigilant about your health. Working with your doctor, you should develop strategies to keep blood glucose at healthy target levels. Over the course of your pregnancy, you may need to increase your insulin dosage to keep up with increased insulin resistance from the hormones of pregnancy. By the third trimester, some women may even have to double or triple the amount of insulin they take.

You should also consult a registered dietitian about healthy eating habits. The dietitian can help you determine a caloric intake that will allow you to gain a healthy amount of weight without gaining too much. You may be advised to eat several small meals a day to help you stabilize blood glucose levels and avoid morning sickness.

If you were fit before pregnancy, you will be encouraged to continue exercising. Regular exercise helps control blood glucose levels and prepares you for the rigors of labor and delivery. Do not start a strenuous new workout now, but do try to get some exercise even if you didn't exercise before. You should talk to your doctor before starting any exercise regimen.

During your pregnancy, be sure to closely monitor your blood glucose several times a day: before and after meals, at bedtime, and in the middle of the night. Monitoring will help you determine whether you need to adjust insulin dosages. It can also help you detect hypoglycemia. Some pregnant women develop hypoglycemia unawareness and can no longer tell if they are having a bout of low blood sugar. Hypoglycemia can be very dangerous to the mother and may lead to seizures.

Challenges of Labor and Delivery
Once you go into labor, your doctor will continuously monitor your blood glucose level to make sure it is as close to normal as possible. Because you may need a caesarean section, you will not be allowed to eat, a fact that can make glucose control more difficult. Instead, you will be given an intravenous catheter to supply you with the energy you need, should the labor be prolonged. Most women do not need insulin during labor, but it is available intravenously, if needed.

Birth and Pregnancy Complications
Women who have diabetes may face complications in their pregnancies. Among them:

Macrosomia

During pregnancy, the fetus gets all its nutrients from the mother's blood. If that blood contains too much glucose, the fetus's pancreas goes into overdrive to produce extra insulin to use up that glucose. So while the mother may not be able to manufacture enough insulin, the fetus can do this on its own.

But rather than burn it up for energy, the glucose is converted into fat, which causes your baby to grow larger and fatter in the womb. The result is macrosomia, which literally means large body. A baby with macrosomia is at greater risk for delivery by caesarean section. In some cases, the baby needs to be delivered early. Large babies delivered early are at greater risk for having health problems such as respiratory distress because the lungs are not mature yet.

Preeclampsia

Women with diabetes are at greater risk for developing preeclampsia, also called toxemia, a condition in which blood pressure gets too high. The condition produces several symptoms including swelling in your feet and lower legs, and leaking of protein into your urine. You may notice sudden weight gain and develop headaches, nausea, vomiting, abdominal pain, and blurry vision. Preeclampsia is usually detected by a blood pressure check or with a urine test. The condition is very serious and if untreated, can cause seizures, coma, and death to you or your baby.

If you are diagnosed with preeclampsia, you may be confined to bed rest for the duration of your pregnancy. However, the only real cure is delivery. Your doctor will help you keep an eye out for preeclampsia by regularly monitoring your blood pressure. You may be asked to take your own blood pressure at home. Your OB/GYN may also examine you and the baby to determine whether a premature delivery is viable. If so, the baby will probably be delivered by caesarean section.

Hypoglycemia

A baby born to a mother with diabetes is at risk for experiencing hypoglycemia immediately after delivery. If the mother's blood sugar has been consistently high during the pregnancy, the baby will have high levels of insulin in circulation. After delivery, the high insulin levels persist, but the baby no longer has the high level of sugar coming from its mother. As a result, the newborn's blood sugar will fall to lower levels. Close monitoring in the first twenty-four hours is usually required. If the baby's blood glucose levels get too low, intravenous doses of glucose may be necessary.

Jaundice

Another risk for babies born to diabetic mothers is jaundice, a condition that can also occur in babies born to women without diabetes. During gestation, your baby produces large amounts of red blood cells that are no longer needed after delivery. The red blood cells are then broken down, a process that produces bilirubin. The bilirubin is then processed by the liver and eliminated.

If the baby's liver isn't mature enough, the process cannot be accomplished, and the bilirubin lingers in the baby, producing a yellowish hue in the baby's skin. The yellow coloring is called jaundice. The condition is usually treated in the hospital by placing the baby under special lights that eliminate the bilirubin.

After the Baby Is Born

The postpartum period poses another set of challenges for women with diabetes. Immediately after delivery, your blood glucose levels may be lower than normal, and you may not need insulin. Sometimes, even women with Type 1 diabetes don't need insulin for several days. It may be a month or two before you resume your prepregnancy diabetes care.

If you choose to breastfeed, you may be lowering the risk of your baby developing diabetes. Studies have found that babies who are breastfed for at least three months have a lower incidence of Type 1 diabetes. When you do breastfeed, be sure to keep a high-carb snack or drink of juice nearby to help you avoid a sudden dip in blood glucose.

In some women, breastfeeding actually makes it easier to control blood glucose. The extra energy burned while nursing allows them to eat more and still not use insulin. But in some women, breastfeeding can cause blood glucose levels to swing as the body produces breastmilk. Be on the lookout for changes in your blood glucose, and consult your physician about ways to help stabilize it. You should not use oral diabetes medication if you choose to breastfeed.

If you manage to find the energy to have sex after the baby is born, be aware that breastfeeding is not a substitute for birth control. Even without resuming your period, you can still get pregnant, and so should still use an effective form of contraception.

Having a newborn in the house can be exhausting. Sleepless nights, fatigue, and hormonal shifts can make it difficult for you to spot symptoms indicating shifts in blood glucose. That's why monitoring your blood glucose is critical, even in this busy time. A bout of hypoglycemia while you're with the baby can be dangerous, so be sure you stay on top of your blood glucose levels, especially when you're alone or driving. Remember, taking good care of yourself will help you take better care of your baby.

A PERSONAL STORY

Linda

All her life, Linda planned on having children. So when she met her husband Ken and fell in love, she knew that even something like Type 2 diabetes was not going to interfere with that dream. It didn't even matter that Ken had Type 1 diabetes.

Linda, a network engineer, was first diagnosed at age eighteen when a routine physical exam detected glucose in her urine. But the doctor, who worked at a college health clinic, gave her no information on what to do next. With no guidance, Linda did nothing.

Six years later, Linda went on a two-month trip through Europe, stopping at a hospital in Turkey to get treatment for a bladder infection. "The doctor said, 'Do you know you have diabetes?' and I said, 'Yeah, I've heard that before,'" recalls Linda, who is now forty. At a hospital in Greece, she decided to get tested and found out that she had blood glucose levels of 500 mg/dl.

Upon her return to the United States, Linda went to see an endocrinologist, who put her on Micronase and later on, Glucophage. Neither medication helped control her blood sugar. Finally, she was put on insulin. "That was really scary, giving myself that first shot," she says. "But you don't realize how bad you feel until you feel good."

Linda eventually got the hang of managing her diabetes, using insulin injections and carb counting. When she met her husband Ken in the early 1990s, it was the first time Linda had encountered another diabetic. 'My mom said, 'What are you doing dating a diabetic?'" Linda says. "But I think it's good because you both know what you're going through." The two of them were soon married.

Because they both had diabetes, they knew that having children was going to be a challenge, both for Linda and the unborn child. But the couple was not deterred, even after they had genetic counseling that told them the chances for having kids with the disease were high.

"The odds of having kids with diabetes are definitely increased with the two of us," Linda says. "But it wasn't a death sentence. The desire to have a complete family with children was more important than dealing with diabetes. Plus, there's always the chance for a cure."

With plans to undertake what Linda calls the most important project of her life, she went ahead and got pregnant. Her blood sugars were already in good control, thanks to her vigilance and commitment, but Linda became even more intensive with her therapy. She checked her blood glucose levels ten times a day, made sure to eat plenty of dark leafy greens and drank a lot of water. She also continued to exercise, taking aerobics, kickboxing, and water aerobics classes. Amazingly, she had HbA1C levels that hovered around five.

But unlike most pregnant women, Linda was at the doctors more frequently during her pregnancy. In addition to her endocrinologist, and regular obstetrician/gynecologist, she also saw another OB/GYN who specialized in high-risk pregnancies. By the end of her pregnancy, she was getting ultrasounds every week, which she considered a rare bonus of having diabetes.

Her need for insulin increased dramatically during her pregnancy as the baby grew. The week before she delivered, Linda had a severe hypoglycemic episode during her water aerobics class. She had checked her blood glucose before she got in the pool and eaten a small snack. Everything appeared fine. But midway through class, her blood sugars plummeted. Linda began blowing bubbles in the pool. When a nurse tried to give her a shot, Linda started screaming.

"I was so out of it," Linda says. "I remember I had to pee, and they wouldn't let me. Finally, in the ride in the ambulance, I remember a woman saying, 'I think her blood sugar is coming back because she's a lot nicer now.'" Looking back, Linda says she thinks that as she approached delivery, her insulin needs dropped, which she didn't expect to happen.

A week after her bout of hypoglycemia, her doctors decided to induce the baby, for fear he'd get too big. Linda gave birth, by vaginal delivery, to Danny, a healthy eight-pound, nine-ounce boy. When she got pregnant again the second time, she was just as vigilant, though she had less time for exercise. Her second child, Rebecca, now almost three, was delivered by caesarean section and also weighed exactly eight pounds and nine ounces.

Looming in the back of her mind is always the concern that her children will develop diabetes someday. She has already had Danny, now four, tested for the autoimmune antibodies that predict diabetes. The results were negative. When Rebecca turns three, she will undergo the same tests. "It's one of my biggest fears that they'll have diabetes," Linda says. "But it didn't stop us from having kids."

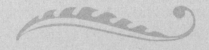

CHAPTER TWELVE 🖋

The Emotional Impact of Diabetes

A chronic disease that affects virtually every aspect of your life is undoubtedly going to take a toll at some point on your emotional and mental well-being. You may feel angry initially when you get the diagnosis. You may experience stress as you struggle to raise your children, hold a job, and manage your diabetes. You may feel overwhelmed at the enormity of the disease and the complexities involved in taking care of your health. Some days, you may simply wind up feeling sad about having diabetes.

Your emotional well-being can have a direct impact on how well you manage your diabetes and how well your blood sugars are controlled. That's why it's important for you to pay attention to your emotional state. You may find you need the help of a mental health professional to get you over a difficult period. Consider mental health another part of taking care of yourself as you deal with diabetes.

Depression
It should come as no surprise that people who have diabetes are prone to depression. After all, the rigors of managing the disease are extensive

and can involve everything from eliminating favorite foods from your diet to self-administering painful injections of insulin. Left unmanaged, diabetes can spiral out of control, causing debilitating complications that can affect all aspects of your health.

Depression is a serious disorder that impairs the way you function. As much as 9.5 percent of the population or nearly nineteen million people suffer from a depressive illness every year. The condition can destroy a person's career, family life, and other relationships and cause enormous pain and suffering.

Among people with diabetes, there is generally a greater likelihood for developing depression, though it's not clear whether depression results from the stress of having diabetes or diabetes is causing metabolic changes in the brain. According to one study, the incidence of depression among diabetics may be as much as double that of healthy people. Other studies have shown that having Type 2 diabetes is an indicator for depression. Depression may also be a predictor of poor health in diabetics. In a study of older Mexican Americans published in *Diabetes Care,* those who had depression were more likely to have complications from diabetes, ranging from cardiovascular problems to nephropathy, neuropathy, and retinopathy. That's why depression needs to be taken seriously and treated promptly.

How Depression Affects Diabetes

People who have depression along with diabetes are less likely to take good care of their health. They may eat more than they should and not pay attention to the foods they choose, causing them to gain weight, which only fuels their misery. Or they may not eat enough and risk hypoglycemia. People who become depressed are also less likely to adhere to their insulin regimen and take their medications properly. They may be less compliant with monitoring their blood glucose and less interested in getting regular exercise.

As you can see, depression can affect how well blood glucose is controlled. If blood glucose goes out of control, you may experience more fatigue and sleepiness, which only heightens your depressive symptoms. In addition, the elevated blood glucose levels will raise your risk for diabetic complications.

A Case of the Blues or Depression?

It isn't always easy to determine whether you're experiencing a bout of sadness or a serious case of depression. After all, most people suffer from an occasional case of the blues, and being told you have diabetes is certainly enough to make even the most jovial person feel sad. But according to the National Institute of Mental Health, there are some telltale signs of serious depression:

- Persistent, sad, anxious, or empty mood.
- Feelings of hopelessness and pessimism.
- Feelings of guilt, worthlessness, and helplessness.
- Loss of interest or pleasure in hobbies and activities you once enjoyed, including sex.
- Decreased energy, fatigue, and feeling slowed down.
- Difficulty concentrating, remembering, or making decisions.
- Insomnia, early awakening, or oversleeping.
- Appetite changes or fluctuations in weight.
- Thoughts of death or suicide, or suicide attempts.
- Restlessness or irritability.

If you have five or more of these symptoms every day for at least two weeks, and they begin to interfere with your daily living, you should be evaluated for depression.

Treating Diabetics with Depression

Suffering from depression while you have diabetes can be a dangerous combination. Depression can impact your ability to care for your health, making you less inclined to eat well, exercise, or take your insulin or medications.

If you're experiencing more than a mild case of the blues, you may need professional treatment. Some physical disorders, such as thyroid disease, anemia, or a neurological disorder can cause depressive symptoms. Occasionally, a medication can bring on symptoms of depression.

The treatment of depression must be tailored to the individual and may involve pharmaceuticals, psychotherapy, or a combination of both. Before seeking any treatment, you should consult with a mental-health professional who is trained to diagnose your condition. Possible drug treatments include:

- *Selective serotonin reuptake inhibitors (SSRIs).* These medications work by blocking the removal of serotonin, a neurotransmitter involved in regulating mood, in the synapses, or gaps between the nerves. Inadequate amounts of serotonin, as well as other neurotransmitters such as dopamine and norepinephrine are often the cause of depression. In recent years, these drugs have become enormously popular as the medication of choice for treating depression. Common drugs include fluoxetine (Prozac), paroxetine (Paxil), escitalopram (Lexapro), and sertraline (Zoloft). Possible side effects include jitteryness, headache, nervousness, insomnia, and sexual problems.
- *Tricyclics.* These drugs work by restoring chemical imbalances in the brain that can cause depression. Although initially introduced to treat depression, they are also used to reduce the symptoms of panic attacks, post-traumatic stress disorder, and obsessive compulsive disorder. Among the drugs in this category are amitriptyline (Elavil), clomipramine (Anafril), imipramine pamoate (Tofranil PM), and nortriptyline (Aventyle). These medications generally have more side effects than the SSRIs, including dry mouth, constipation, and blurred vision.

- *Monoamine oxidase inhibitors (MAOIs).* Because these medications require dietary restrictions, doctors are more likely to try other antidepressants first. Certain cheeses and wines are contraindicated because they contain a substance called tyramine, which, combined with MAOIs, can cause extremely high blood pressure. Nasal decongestants can cause similar problems. The drugs in this category are generally used to treat panic disorder, social phobia, PTSD, and sometimes OCD. Drugs in this category are isoarboxazid (Marplan), phenelzine (Nardil), and tranylcypromine (Parnate).
- *Other antidepressants.* Some drugs used to treat depression don't share the same chemical structure with one another, but share the same goal of stabilizing the chemicals in the brain, namely serotonin, norephinephrine, and dopamine. Drugs in this loosely organized category include buproprion (Wellbutrin), venlafaxine (Effexor), and mirtazapine (Remeron). Lithium, which also belongs in this group, is more commonly used to treat manic-depressive symptoms.

What About Psychotherapy?

Maybe you'd rather talk to someone about your depression. Some people may benefit from psychotherapy. By talking problems through with a trained therapist, patients can overcome their depression. Sometimes, the therapy may focus on the problematic relationships in the patient's life that are exacerbating the depression, known as interpersonal therapy. Another kind, cognitive-behavioral therapy, works to help the patient change the way he thinks and behaves in order to reduce depression.

Only by working with your mental-health professional can you determine the best course of treatment for your depression. Professionals trained to deal with mental-health issues include psychiatrists, psychologists, licensed social workers, psychiatric nurses, and mental-health counselors. The most important thing to realize is that depression has a very direct impact on your diabetes. It can cause high blood glucose that brings symptoms similar to those of depression, including fatigue and sleepiness. It can also interfere with your desire and ability to manage the disease, which will jeopardize your health in the long run.

Stress

Everyone experiences different levels of stress, depending on life circumstances and how you interpret them. Some people may find the morning commute a stressful experience, while others may enjoy the solace and find no discomfort traveling on busy roads. Some people may find holiday shopping stressful. Others may take great joy in it. In people who have diabetes, there's a great likelihood for stress, given the high maintenance it requires to manage the disease. Too much stress however, can have a direct effect on the disease itself, usually by worsening the diabetes.

When the body experiences stress, it responds as if under attack. Stress might be caused by a major crisis in your life like a devastating illness, problems with your finances, or troubles in your marriage. Or it might be something less traumatic, like a fight with your spouse, rushing late to an appointment, or forgetting to pay a bill on time. Stress is also caused by physical injury, such as illness or surgery. Even happy events can cause stress, such as an upcoming party or a job promotion.

In any case, stress causes your body to go into a fight-or-flight response, as it prepares to take action in response to the stress. Hormone levels shoot up, causing stored energy in your cells to become more available. This stored energy is in the form of fat and glucose, and is made available to help you flee the imminent danger. But if there is nothing to actually run from—as is the case when the stress is primarily in your mind—then the excess energy stores go unused, causing blood glucose levels to go up.

Stress can also affect blood glucose levels in another way. When you're under stress, you're less likely to do a good job of managing your diabetes. You may drink more alcohol, eat more unhealthy foods, and skip your exercise routine. You may forget to monitor your blood sugar and skip an insulin injection or medication.

How to Manage Stress

While it might be hard to escape the drain of working for a nasty boss or the exhaustion of caring for elderly parents, there are steps you can take to minimize the stress that these situations can cause. Some good tips to keep in mind:

- *Replace bad thoughts with good ones.* Sometimes, simply fine tuning the way you think about a situation can make all the difference. For instance, say you hate your job. You may not be able to leave it as soon as you'd like but you can change the way you look at it. Maybe you have good friends in the office or you enjoy the short commute. Perhaps you like the work you do. Whatever it is, try to see the positives, even in a bad situation.
- *Take steps toward change.* Don't sit back and passively allow events to occur. Taking action toward change can help alleviate your stress. So if you're stressed out over your marriage, consider seeking marital counseling. If it's your job you can't stand, launch a job search or consider a career change. If you're over-whelmed with credit card debt, consider buying everything with cash only from now on or cutting up your cards. By taking active steps to change your situation, you will feel more in control and less helpless.
- *Enlist the help of others.* If certain circumstances are making you stressed out, you might want to find other people to help you. Perhaps having diabetes has become simply too stressful. Try looking for a support group, where you can meet others in your situation. Or if it's caring for elderly parents that has you stressed, look for caregivers who can fill in for you on occasion.

If you simply want to vent about your stressors, call a good friend and air your gripes. Simply having the support of other people can help you feel less stressed.

- *Practice relaxation.* Making time to relax in your busy day can help lessen the impact of stress. You might consider learning to meditate, doing yoga, or practicing breathing exercises. Taking a walk in nature can also help you relax. And in moments of stress, try reciting a favorite prayer, poem, or quote that you find calming.
- *Incorporate pleasurable activities into your day.* Go back to a favorite hobby or sport you once enjoyed, and lose yourself in it. Watch a favorite movie or television sitcom. Doing something you love for even a short period can help you feel less stressed.
- *Seek professional help if necessary.* If you find stress has become overwhelming, consider discussing it with a mental health professional. You may need to take more aggressive steps to reduce your stress, especially if it's taking a toll on your care.

Other Harmful Emotions

Being diagnosed with diabetes and having the disease can spur a range of emotions. Depression and stress are just two of those. Other feelings you might experience can also affect your health and well-being. These include anger and denial.

Denial

You do not want to admit that you have a chronic disease, so you tell yourself it's okay if you eat just one more bite, postpone a sorely needed visit to your doctor, or convince yourself that the infection on your foot is nothing serious. Any time you try to deny that something bad could happen or is happening, you risk not caring for your health and managing your disease.

If you have no symptoms, it may be especially easy to deny you have an illness. In fact, it may be a way for you to cope with the devastating news that you have diabetes. So you go about your routine and pay no attention to your health, doing little to take care of your diabetes. You continue to eat an unhealthy diet, you say you have no time to exercise, and you convince yourself that a couple of drinks is okay. But living in denial for too long can jeopardize your health if you neglect your diabetes.

What to Do

Getting rid of the denial may not be easy. It helps to start by learning about the disease and finding out what you need to do to stay healthy. Once you've educated yourself, set some health goals. Maybe you want to lose weight. Perhaps you want to start exercising. Or maybe you need to devise an eating plan. Enlist the help of trained professionals to help you reach your goals as well as family and friends who can offer their support. By taking control of your situation, you will become an active player in your health and well-being..

Anger

Perhaps you are outraged that you have diabetes, especially if you've been taking care of yourself all along. You might feel angry about the frequent blood glucose checks and the routine visits to the pharmacy that interfere with your busy schedule. Anger over something you can't control is a normal emotion, one you're likely to experience when you have diabetes. The constant presence of threats to your health can make you feel that life is unfair.

If you find yourself frequently angry, try to determine the source of your anger. Maybe it's the feelings of helplessness. Or maybe you hate the way you can't eat as much at a holiday party. Perhaps you don't like feeling different from other people.

Use your anger to help you take control of your situation. Talk to a counselor about your feelings. Seek out a dietitian and find out ways to enjoy a little extra food without compromising your health. Consider joining a support group with other diabetics that will help you feel less isolated.

Getting Support from Family and Friends

One of the most important things diabetics can do is to seek out support from friends. There will be days when you need nothing more than a compassionate ear to help you get through a frustrating week of maintaining your blood glucose level. Or maybe you simply need a friend to accompany you on healthy walks on a nearby nature trail. Perhaps you will need a neighbor to go with you on a particularly worrisome visit to a doctor's office.

Find family members and friends who are especially supportive and available. Don't dismiss your troubles as insignificant or tedious. People who truly care about you will make themselves available to help you through every challenge you face, from the most minor events to the most serious crises.

Support Groups

Finding support from the people who love you most will really help you as you go through the rigors of managing your disease. But sometimes, they simply cannot understand everything that is involved in having diabetes. It's hard to know exactly what it's like to experience hypoglycemia, administer an insulin injection, or to practice carbohydrate counting at every single meal. That's why you might want to consider joining a support group.

Talk to your doctor about support groups in your area. Or consider going on-line to find people who are in the same predicament. Sharing your problems with others who know exactly what you're going through can help you get past tough periods.

A Final Note

Sir William Osler was a great internist who was once quoted as saying: "If you want to live a long life, develop a chronic disease, and take good care of it." There's no doubt that that's true of diabetes. Taking care of diabetes is a lot like learning to ride a bike. It is a lot of hard work initially, but it does get easier, and you can eventually cruise along without thinking about every turn or maneuver.

But along the way, diabetes can take an emotional toll, too. Having a chronic disease that requires enormous amounts of maintenance isn't easy on anyone and will require great strength and courage on your part. By accepting and working through the complex feelings that can arise, you can take charge of your emotional health. When you're able to overcome depression, anger, and denial, you'll be better equipped to take care of your physical health and live a happier life.

CHAPTER THIRTEEN 🌿

When Your Child Has Diabetes

Parenting isn't an easy job for anyone. On top of raising children who will become good people, we want our children to be healthy, eat well, exercise, and learn to take care of themselves. But when your child's health is complicated by diabetes, you will face challenges that go well beyond the norm.

At birthday parties, your little child may rebel against your restrictions on eating too much cake. She may balk at your insistence that she exercise every day. As a teenager, she may refuse to do routine blood glucose checks or become negligent about administering enough insulin.

Raising children with diabetes is no doubt a monumental feat, but it's not impossible. There are thousands of other parents like you who are already juggling homework and birthday parties with insulin injections and carb counting. But like any challenge of parenting, it will require discipline and perseverance on your part.

When You Get the Diagnosis

Maybe you already suspected your child had diabetes. Symptoms such as thirst and frequent urination made it obvious that something was wrong. Knowing someone in your family had it might have raised your suspicions even more.

But now the doctor has confirmed your greatest fear: Your child has diabetes.

The news may overwhelm you. You may experience feelings of fear, sadness, guilt, and anger. Why your child? How will you ever help her live with this disease? How will this affect the rest of your family?

Once the news sinks in, there's no time to waste. You need to take action to get educated and start teaching your child the rigors of managing diabetes. In the process, you'll discover that your child can still live a normal life with the disease. Here's what you need to do:

- *Learn everything you can about diabetes.* The more you know, the more confident you'll become at managing this disease and passing on your knowledge to your child. Do your own research in the library and on the Internet, using resources such as the American Diabetes Association, the Juvenile Diabetes Foundation, and the National Institute of Diabetes and Digestive and Kidney Diseases of the National Institutes of Health. Get familiar with the day-to-day strategies for keeping blood glucose levels in check, but also learn about emergencies like hypoglycemia and how to handle them.
- *Assemble a medical team.* You may already have a pediatrician or primary care doctor who has taken care of your child for years, but you may need others to help now that your child has been diagnosed with diabetes. Other people to involve include:
  - ~ *An endocrinologist,* who specializes in treating children with diabetes.
  - ~ *A registered dietitian* (RD), who can help you create a meal plan that is kid-friendly. The dietitian should also help you learn to practice ways to control your child's carbohydrate intake, with tools like carb counting. Ask her for tips on

how toc ook a meal for an entire family that is also healthy for your diabetic child.

~ *A certified diabetes educator (CDE),* who can teach you how to manage the day-to-day routines of balancing food intake with insulin and activity. A CDE can also help you find other resources and information about caring for your child's health.

~ *The school nurse,* who will be involved in your child's care at school. Make sure the nurse knows about the diagnosis and understands the demands of caring for a diabetic child. Remember, the school nurse will be an important ally in your child's health care.

• *Look for ways to involve your child in taking care of herself without compromising her care.* Obviously, if your child is only two, she will be too young to get involved in doing her own blood glucose checks. But if your child is school-aged, she may be able to do her own checks and even administer her own insulin. You can also involve your child in making healthy food choices and decisions on exercise activities. Getting your child involved now will empower her and give her the sense of control she'll need for a lifetime.

• *Stick to a regular schedule of eating.* Erratic eating can make it difficult to control blood sugars. By eating snacks and meals at the same time every day, you can help your child maintain a more controlled schedule, which makes it easier to control her blood glucose levels.

• *Get your child active.* Regular exercise is important to helping your child regulate blood glucose levels. So whether it's a sports team, an exercise class, or a romp at the local playground, the key is for your child to move her body. And getting her in the habit now, at a young age, will help her make it a part of her life in the future.

- *Try to be matter-of-fact about the diagnosis and disease.* Having diabetes today is not as serious as it once was. The Joslin Diabetes Clinic in Boston used to give out twenty-five-year awards, then forty, and now fifty-year awards to patients who lived that many years beyond the onset of Type 1 diabetes. If you try to take the news and condition in stride, your child will be more likely to react the same way. She'll come to accept the rigors of managing her condition simply as part of her everyday routine.
- *Make sure everyone around your child is familiar with her condition.* Babysitters, caregivers, grandparents, and others who spend a lot of time with your child should also know how to check your child's blood glucose, give an insulin injection, and spot the signs of hypoglycemia. They should know exactly what to do in the event of an emergency.
- *Look for sources of support within the family and in the community.* A support group for parents of children with diabetes can help you air your fears and concerns, and help you feel less isolated.
- *Take care of yourself, and your marriage, too.* Managing your child's diabetes is a full-time occupation, one that demands enormous patience. Giving yourself an occasional respite will help you recharge and make you a better parent. And if you're married, be sure to take time for you and your spouse. Diabetes can overwhelm a family.

Don't Get Too Intense

While attaining blood glucose levels that are as close to normal as possible is a good goal for most adults, in children under seven it might not be a good idea. Tightly regulated blood glucose can put your child at risk for hypoglycemia, and children this young are usually not able to tell the symptoms. A severe case of recurrent, prolonged hypoglycemia can interfere with a child's normal brain development if seizures are involved.

If you do want to practice intensive management, make sure to do it with caution and under a doctor's close supervision.

Honeymoon Over Already?

In some patients who have Type 1 diabetes, the beta cells will frequently recover some function after a patient starts insulin, which allows for a more stable period of up to four to five years after the initial diagnosis. This is called a honeymoon phase. While this may be good news for awhile, be sure to stay on top of your child's care and remain in close contact with the endocrinologist. Unfortunately, it's short-lived.

Diabetes through the Ages

The way your child responds to having diabetes will depend in part on her temperament, but also on her age. Toddlers are too young to understand the disease, and parents and caregivers will have to do all the work, saying simply that the shots and glucose monitoring are meant to keep them healthy. Preschoolers may ask a lot of questions as they try to comprehend their condition. Any explanation should be kept short and simple, in terms your child understands.

Once she reaches the school years, your child will begin to understand what the disease is and what's involved in taking care of it. You should always follow your child's lead on how much care she can handle on her own. Not every child will be able or interested to do blood glucose checks or administer insulin injections. But some might prefer the feeling of competence that comes with self-care. Whatever your child chooses, make sure you remain involved. It will take awhile before your child gets the hang of managing diabetes.

Over the summer, consider sending your child to a diabetes camp. Time spent at diabetes camp can be one of the best experiences a child or teenager can have. They will see that many other children have the disease and begin to learn how to deal with it. Parents also get a much needed break.

With the onset of the teen years, your child may grow frustrated by the demands of being a diabetic. She may resent feeling different and start to rebel against parental rules, even ones that have direct effects on her health. Parents can help by keeping their teen informed about the consequences and rewards of the choices they make. Even worse, blood glucose control may become more difficult to achieve as hormones increase.

Special issues may arise during these turbulent years. Drinking alcohol, using drugs, and having sex may all become part of the life of your teenager. Beware too that some girls may neglect taking insulin as a way to control their weight. All these behaviors can have an impact on your child's diabetes. Be sure your child knows how these behaviors can harm her health. Encourage her to continue to stay on top of her diabetes.

Working with the School

Communication is key when it comes to addressing your child's diabetes in school. It will be up to you to make sure your child's diabetes is properly monitored and cared for during the hours spent in school. You should meet with your child's teacher, the school nurse, and the principal to discuss your child's condition. Remember, only 1 in 500 children have Type 1 diabetes, and the school may not have a lot of experience with hypoglycemia and the timing of snacks. Things they need to know include:

- *Blood glucose monitoring.* When should they monitor your child's blood glucose? How often? Are there times when we should do extra checks? What is her target range?
- *Meals and snacks.* When should your child eat a snack? Does she usually need a snack after exercise? Are there foods your child should avoid? Can your child do her own carb counting? Is she likely to follow the meal plan you have given her?

- *Exercise.* Are there restrictions on her activities? What can she be given in the event she needs a quick source of glucose? Should she not exercise if her blood glucose is below or above a certain level?
- *Insulin.* What kind does she take? How much does she need? What time? Does she need a shot during the school day? Can she give herself a shot? How much should be given if blood glucose levels are high or low? If she has a pump, can she manage it and do any troubleshooting that's required?
- *Emergency care.* Has your child had hypoglycemia before? What are the signs and symptoms? What should be done to treat it? Does the school need to be provided with glucagon or fast-acting glucose? What are the signs and symptoms that your child has hyperglycemia? How should hyperglycemia be treated?

There are also things that you should find out from the school:

- Who is in charge of your child's care there? Is there a nurse on duty to tend to her? Who will tend to her if she goes on a field trip?
- What time will your child eat lunch? When will she have snacks?
- When does your child have gym class? Can she be excused if her blood glucose is too high or too low?
- Where will your child's food and medical emergency supplies be kept?

Finally, be sure the school has the correct contact information for you and your spouse—phone numbers for home and office, and your cell phone numbers. The school should also have the names and numbers of your child's pediatrician, endocrinologist, and any other emergency contacts, such as relatives living nearby.

Your Child's Rights in School

No child with diabetes should be subject to discrimination or anything less than fair treatment in school, according to federal laws that protect people with disabilities. Schools are required to provide the services that children with disabilities need and to accommodate their unique health needs.

So your child should be able to eat whenever necessary, receive assistance with blood glucose checks and insulin injections, use the bathroom and water fountain whenever needed, and refrain from exercise if blood glucose levels are too low or high. Your child should also be able to participate in any activity that other children do, including field trips, social events, and extracurricular activities. In addition, your child should be permitted extra absences if she is sick or needs to go to a doctor's appointment.

The Surge in Type 2 Diabetes

Until recent years, virtually all children who were diagnosed with diabetes were told they had Type 1 diabetes. Type 2 diabetes was a condition that occurred with advancing age. Not so anymore. In the last twenty years, the number of children being diagnosed with Type 2 diabetes has increased dramatically, enough to cause major concern among public health officials.

Specific numbers are hard to get, but experts estimate that 8 to 45 percent of all kids with newly diagnosed diabetes have Type 2, depending on how the sampling was done and the ethnic makeup of the children. Type 2 diabetes is more prevalent among overweight children and those from certain ethnic groups, including African Americans, Hispanic Americans, Asian Americans, and Native Americans.

Most children who have Type 2 diabetes are over the age of ten and are in mid-to-late puberty, though children as young as four have been diagnosed. Many of them come from families with a history of diabetes. In fact, 45 to 80 percent of the children with Type 2 diabetes have at least one parent with the same disease.

The increasing numbers of children with Type 2 diabetes comes at a time when more and more children are overweight. The weight gain is perpetuated by unhealthy diets and snacks, often eaten on the run or in fast-food restaurants. Compounding the problem is the lack of regular exercise as more children spend their free time in front of the television or computer instead of engaging in physical activity. By some estimates, approximately 11 percent of all children are clinically overweight.

Type 2 diabetes is also more common in girls than boys, a fact that leads some experts to wonder whether hormones are involved. The disease is usually diagnosed in mid-puberty, when growth hormones may be promoting insulin resistance.

Can Type 2 Diabetes Be Prevented?

At the rate we are going, the CDC predicts that one in three children born in the year 2000 will go on to develop diabetes at some point in their lives. That's a frightening prediction on many levels. People who are diagnosed at an early age will have a greater likelihood for developing complications simply because they have more time to do so. The disease will also exact a huge economic toll on the national budget.

The only hope we have is to intervene by making lifestyle changes in our children—the same ones that help protect adults from developing Type 2 diabetes. These are:

- *Limit foods with empty calories and encourage healthy eating.* It isn't easy to coax a young child who prefers high-fat sweets and fried foods to eat healthy fruits, vegetables, and whole-grain foods. But a diet rich in these foods can help your child lose weight. It will also help establish healthy eating habits that will last a lifetime.
- *Keep an eye on portion sizes.* Don't allow your child to overeat. Encourage her to stop eating when she's full. Avoid piling too much food on her plate and then telling her to eat it all.
- *Encourage exercise.* Dietary changes alone will not be enough to turn the tide, so get your child involved in activities that make

her active. If your child prefers competitive sports, enroll her on a team. If she's less inclined toward athletics, consider taking her on walks, hiking, or snowshoeing. Even simple games of tag, riding a scooter, or playing on swings can help. Ideally, your child should get thirty minutes of activity a day.

- *Look for ways to incorporate activity into daily routines.* Consider walking to school instead of taking the bus. Walk the long way to the store in the mall. Take the stairs, not the elevator. The same strategies to get adults more active will work with children, too.
- *Help your child lose weight.* If your child is overweight, employing these strategies will help her shed the extra pounds that could put her at risk for developing diabetes. Talk to your pediatrician about a healthy weight goal and ways you can ensure your child maintains a healthy weight.

Your Child's Future

Although you may be plagued with fears and worries about your child's future as a diabetic, there are numerous examples of people who have gone on to live long, productive lives, even after a diagnosis of diabetes. Consider actress Mary Tyler Moore, who has battled tirelessly on behalf of the Juvenile Diabetes Research Foundation, former Miss America of 1999 Nicole Johnson, retired baseball player Dave Hollins, and lead vocalist Bret Michaels of the rock band Poison. The lesson you can learn from their example—and thousands of lesser known people with the disease—is this: A diagnosis of diabetes does not and should not diminish your child's goals, dreams, and ambitions. Diabetes may be a nuisance to manage, but it should never be an impediment to your child's abilities to fulfill her dreams.

PERSONAL STORIES

Jenny

Having a child with diabetes is never easy. But Jenny, a forty-year-old mother, has two kids with Type 1 diabetes: Amanda, twelve and a half years old, and Ryan, eight and a half years old.

Amanda, was diagnosed at the age of four, seven months after she had Coxsackie virus. Like most diabetics, her first symptoms were excessive thirst and frequent urination. But Jenny knew nothing of diabetes and had no idea why her daughter was drinking so much. It wasn't until she went to a doctor and had her blood glucose tested that they learned Amanda had diabetes.

Fearful that her son Ryan would have diabetes too, Jenny and her husband CJ took Ryan to the Joslin Center in Boston for genetic testing. The tests came back negative. But not long after their trip to Boston, Amanda noticed that her little brother, then three, was drinking a lot and urinating more than usual. "To humor her, I said, 'Oh, okay, let's test his blood,'" Jenny says. "But when I did, it was up in the 400s."

Managing diabetes for two young children quickly became a part of Jenny's daily life, and the routine has continued. The children check their blood glucose at least four times a day, with an occasional middle-of-the-night check, if necessary. Amanda wears a pump and sets her own insulin levels, but Ryan still relies on his mother to administer the shots he needs, which are given twice a day. "I always try to do it for them as much as possible," Jenny says. "An endocrinologist once told me, 'They have the rest of their lives to do this stuff.' So I always do it now, whenever I can."

Meals and snacks are served at almost the same time every day, and Jenny guards against doing even the tiniest thing that could throw off her children's blood glucose—from skipping an evening snack to eating a meal too late. She says she can't even imagine what it would be like to have a morning without blood glucose checks, insulin shots, and carb counting.

It took a long time for Jenny to learn the rigors of diabetes management. Until her children were diagnosed, Jenny knew nothing of it and didn't even know that her great grandfather had it in the 1920s. As one of the early patients to receive insulin, he lived another 20 years after his diagnosis, which was considered a long time back then.

In fact, the only thing Jenny knew about diabetes was that people who had it should not eat sugar, a fallacy that has since been shattered by the research behind carbohydrate counting, a tool Jenny uses with her children. Though she had tried the exchange system early on with Amanda, the meals were too limited and didn't include enough foods for children. After an eight-week course with a registered dietitian, Jenny began using carb counting. The technique has given her enormous flexibility in terms of her children's food choices.

"When she was first diagnosed, I thought about Halloween and just cried," Jenny says. "When we got into carb counting, I realized we could still have Halloween."

Jenny also learned the hard way about hypoglycemia. When Amanda was just five years old, she came downstairs one night, screaming at the top of her lungs. "She just kept screaming, 'I love you, mommy. I love you, daddy. Help me, help me!'" Jenny recalls. "She was literally losing her mind."

Still relatively inexperienced, Jenny and CJ had no idea what was going on. When they realized it, they were terrified and struggled with trembling hands to figure out how to use the glucagon. By the time Amanda was injected, her blood glucose was still only at 20 mg/dl.

Looking back, Jenny knows exactly what she did wrong: Amanda had eaten a late dinner and had a smaller than normal snack that night. "I just thought she was going to be okay," Jenny says. "I should have checked before she went to bed." Amanda has since had only one other episode, while Ryan, who has benefited from the experience of his older sister, has not had hypoglycemia.

Right from the start, Jenny was determined not to let diabetes interfere with her children's lives. She and CJ also decided that being active was going to be a critical part of their lives. "We knew that the more active they were, the healthier they would be," she says.

As a result, the children are both skilled soccer players, students of tae kwon do—Amanda has a black belt—and avid waterskiers, swimmers, and skiers. In fact, Amanda was just recently accepted to the state's Olympic Development Program in soccer.

Both children excel academically and juggle busy social lives despite the frequent blood glucose checks and need for insulin injections. Jenny has also gotten her children involved in lobbying efforts to secure more funding for research on Type 1 diabetes. Over the years, they have raised $15,000 toward diabetes research.

A couple of years ago, Amanda began using a pump, which has only made it easier for her to manage her diabetes. "She likes the control because she wants to be able to do it herself," Jenny says. "But sometimes, she still forgets to bolus or doesn't bolus enough." She also does her own blood glucose checks.

Having diabetes has also forced Jenny to become a constant presence in the schools, where she always makes a point to get to know the school nurse. The nurses get detailed instructions about her children's diabetes management, and Jenny makes sure to stay in close touch with frequent calls and holiday gifts. So if, for instance, Ryan awakens with high blood glucose, Jenny will give him some extra insulin and alert the school nurse, just to keep her informed.

But all her hard work and positive attitude cannot erase Jenny's constant worries. "Even if you work really hard and you monitor them 24/7, there's always that worry factor," she says. "I always worry that even if I do everything right, it still might not be good enough."

Most days, Jenny can brush those worries aside and focus on all the things her kids are accomplishing in spite of having the disease. "People usually can't even believe they have diabetes," she says. "But I always say, you just can't let it stop you. You can do anything you want. You can still play soccer, and you can still get a black belt. And you can still have diabetes."

Lily

As an Asian-American, Lily already stands out in her predominantly white high school. But as a diabetic, Lily stands out in other ways, too.

In the middle of classes, Lily, sixteen, sometimes has to leave to go check her blood sugar levels when she feels nauseous or shaky. She is sometimes unable to accompany her friends to the mall after school because her blood sugars are off. And she is forever struggling to balance her food intake with her exercise and adjusting her insulin to match.

"It's just such a hassle when you have diabetes," she says. "It's such a high maintenance disease."

Lily was diagnosed at eleven, when she came home from summer camp complaining of excessive thirst. She could down a two-liter bottle of water in a single sitting and still feel thirsty. She also spent the week urinating all through the night. Her mother, a nurse, suspected diabetes immediately. A doctor confirmed her suspicions within twenty-four hours.

Lily reacted with anger at the news. She didn't want to be different from her classmates. No one else at the school had diabetes, and most kids didn't even know what it was. Lily found herself educating her peers constantly, as she explained her visits to the nurse's office and why she sometimes couldn't participate in gym class. "Fortunately, I have good friends who understood right away," she says.

What Lily hated most were the insulin injections. The needle hurt, and a year into her disease, she asked her doctor for a pump. The pump is attached to her abdomen, and Lily wears it like a pager on her belt. She says the pump has definitely made life as a diabetic a lot easier.

What bothers Lily most about having diabetes is the unpredictability of the disease. While on vacation one night, she went to bed with her family, but then didn't wake up the next morning. Unbeknownst to everyone, Lily had developed hypoglycemia overnight, a frightening event that had her parents administering glucagon to revive her.

"Later, my mom figured out that we had gone swimming that night in the hotel pool," Lily says. "I swam maybe a few minutes longer than I should have, and that used up my glucose. And I didn't adjust my night time insulin to make up for the extra exercise because everything seemed normal when I went to bed."

Still, exercise is a critical part of Lily's life. She plays basketball every winter and runs track in the spring. Every chance she gets, she walks to her destination, whether it's a babysitting job or a visit to a friend's house. But always, she monitors her blood glucose afterward to make sure it hasn't gone too low. "It really is a pain," she says.

What has helped is attending a diabetes camp in the summer, where Lily knows she's not alone. She has made some really good friends and learned some valuable ways to take care of her health. During the rest of the year, she and her parents participate in a monthly support group for children with diabetes. The kids come from all over the region, and Lily enjoys the camaraderie.

"Through these other kids and parents, I've come to feel better about having diabetes," Lily says. "My favorite thing has been learning to make some of my own healthy meals. I even serve them to my family now."

CHAPTER FOURTEEN 🌿

The Future of Diabetes

Even while you are wrestling with a diagnosis of diabetes, working out a meal plan, and giving yourself insulin injections, scientists and researchers around the world are working hard to find new ways to treat, detect, and prevent diabetes. Someday, diabetics who are insulin-dependent may no longer need daily injections. Blood glucose levels may be detected by simply applying a patch. A child's likelihood for developing diabetes will be foretold at birth. Someday, there is even hope that diabetes will be cured.

In this final chapter, we'll take a look at some of the research that is underway. Though the research presented here is by no means exhaustive, we hope it will kindle hopes that diabetes will become more manageable, less debilitating, and perhaps even eliminated.

On the Path to a Cure

In an ideal world, diabetes will someday no longer exist, much in the same way scientists have largely eradicated other once formidable diseases like polio, mumps, German measles, and rubella. Research to find a cure is happening in laboratories around the world. Here are just a few promising avenues:

Stem Cell Research

One of the most exciting areas of research involves the use of embryonic stem cells. Some scientists believe that stem cell research may cure several diseases that are triggered by cell destruction, including diabetes, Parkinson's, Alzheimer's, osteoporosis, and multiple sclerosis.

Human embryonic stem cells come from fertilized embryos that are less than a week old. Unlike more mature cells, stem cells are undifferentiated, meaning they have not been assigned a specific task in the body. Scientists have found that these stem cells have the potential to become any other kind of cell, including muscle cells, heart cells, bone cells, and yes, pancreatic beta cells. Research suggests that pancreatic beta cells derived from stem cells may be able to do what regular beta cells do: produce insulin that helps the body use glucose. The beta cells grown from stem cells would then be transplanted into a diabetic to replace the defective cells.

But the research is hindered by several factors. For one thing, scientists say there are not enough stem cells available for research right now. Although present in adult tissue, stem cells that are best suited for growing into other tissues are those found in embryos. Some people believe the use of stem cells for research raises serious moral and ethical questions. After all, human stem cells come from highly charged and controversial sources, namely aborted fetuses, discarded surplus embryos created for in vitro fertilization, and human cloning.

Controversies aside, researchers are hopeful that stem cell research will someday lead to a cure for Type 1 diabetes. Embryonic stem cells from a mouse have already demonstrated the potential for producing insulin. The research on mice may also give clues as to how beta cells are formed.

Islet Cell Transplants

Transplanting islet cells from a healthy pancreas in to people who have diabetes is already underway as an alternative to transplanting the entire pancreas. But the procedure is fraught with challenges caused by transplant rejection, which occurs when the patient's immune system attacks the new islet cells as foreign invaders. Most people who receive islet cells are then required to take large amounts of drugs that suppress their immune systems to prevent this kind of reaction. The problem is, these drugs suppress the entire immune system, making it difficult for the patient to defend himself against even the most minor bacteria and viruses.

In 2000, the hope for success was buoyed by Canadian researchers in a trial called the Edmonton Protocol. Using a glucocorticoid-free immunosuppressive regimen of drugs, researchers were able to reverse insulin dependence in seven patients given islet cell transplants and to sustain that for fourteen months. Efforts to replicate this medical feat are underway.

But even if these efforts are successful, islet cell transplants offer only limited promise. Only about 3,000 pancreases are available every year, and patients typically require islets from two or more pancreases for a successful transplant. Until scientists can develop a ready source of islet cells and successfully address the problems of rejection, this procedure remains uncertain as a cure for Type 1 diabetes.

Regenerating Insulin-Producing Cells

Someday, if current research pans out, diabetics whose beta cells in the pancreas have stopped making insulin may be able to reverse the process and go back to producing insulin. Scientists have isolated a gene that can regenerate insulin-producing cells in the pancreas. The islet neogenesis associated protein, or INGAP, could relieve people who have Type 1 diabetes from the task of administering daily insulin injections and prevent the demise of these insulin-producing cells in Type 2 diabetics. It may also assist in the genetic research that helps identify people who are likely to develop the disease. Currently, clinical trials are underway to determine whether INGAP can help both Type 1 and Type 2 diabetics produce new beta cells.

Liver Cells That Make Insulin

Preliminary research using gene therapy has allowed scientists to convert liver cells into pancreatic cells. Using human cells, scientists selected the same gene that converts stem cells into pancreatic cells, and introduced it to liver cells. Once the gene was introduced, the cells began to grow into pancreatic ones. The newly formed pancreatic cells were even able to produce insulin. But whether the new pancreatic cells will produce insulin in response to glucose and cease to make insulin in its absence remains unknown and will require further research.

New Medications

While some researchers are on the quest for a cure, others are at work trying to improve the way diabetes is treated with new therapies. Many drugs are in various phases of clinical trials, but some are emerging as frontrunners that will someday join sulfonylureas, metformin, and the thiazolinediones as treatment options for people diagnosed with diabetes. These drugs include:

- *Glucagon-like peptide 1 (GLP-1)* hormone may have a role in treating both Type 1 and Type 2 diabetes. The drug has several actions. It stimulates the release of insulin, suppresses the release of the hormone glucagon (which helps release glycogen from the liver when there isn't a supply of food), and slows the digestive process. It also stimulates the growth of new pancreatic beta cells while slowing the death of these cells. Studies show that taken after meals, GLP-1 reduces the amount of blood glucose in patients with Type 1 diabetes. Subcutaneous infusions of GLP-1 lowered the amount of fasting blood glucose in patients with Type 2 diabetes. The hormone works by binding to a receptor on pancreatic beta cells and influencing its insulin-producing actions.

- *Pramlintide acetate (Symlin)* is a synthetic version of the human hormone amylin and first in a class of medications known as amylinomimetic agents or amylin receptor agonists. Like the human form of amylin, Symlin helps in regulating blood glucose. Amylin is produced and secreted in the beta cells of the pancreas and works as a complement to insulin.

  If approved, the treatment will be the first to help control blood glucose in Type 1 diabetics since the discovery of insulin. Symlin would help reduce the surge in glucagon that occurs after meals in both Type 1 and Type 2 diabetics who have come to rely on insulin to control their blood glucose levels. In clinical trials, the drug slowed the rate the stomach empties, reduced the variation in blood glucose levels after a meal and lowered HbA1C levels. Side effects from the use of Symlin were nausea, anorexia, and vomiting

- *Synthetic exendin-4 (Exenatide)* is the first of a new class of medications called incretin mimetic agents. These medications are being developed for Type 2 diabetics who are unable to achieve blood glucose control with lifestyle changes alone. The drug works by stimulating the body's ability to produce insulin in response to higher blood glucose levels, blocking the release of glucagon after a meal, and slowing the rate at which nutrients are absorbed into the bloodstream. In animal studies, Exenatide helped preserve existing beta cells and promoted the formation of new ones.

  In clinical trials, people who used Exenatide experienced reductions in postprandial blood glucose levels. The drug also lowered serum triglyceride levels after a meal. High levels of triglycerides have been associated with a greater risk for cardiovascular disease. In addition, the drug also reduced HbA1C levels. Nausea was the most common side effect associated with Exenatide.

- *Exenatide LAR (long-acting release)* presents the possibility of a once-a-week to once-a-month dosage for a long-acting version of Exenatide. Early studies show that sustained levels of the drug are possible, but more studies are still needed.
- Research is being done on drugs that target the PPAR gamma, or peroxisome proliferator-activated receptor gamma gene. PPAR gamma is a gene that's been identified as a marker for developing Type 2 diabetes. The research shows great promise for identifying people who are at risk for diabetes, but also opens up the opportunity to develop drugs that may have a preventive effect on Type 2 diabetes in obese people.

Type 2 diabetes often requires insulin injections after fifteen years of the disease. This is due to the decline in beta function and apoptosis, or death, of these cells. In animal models, the PPAR gamma medications are showing promise in preventing apoptosis from occurring. Scientists are now studying whether this effect occurs in humans, and results from those studies will be available in the next three years.

In addition to the treatments for diabetes, scientists are exploring exciting new drugs for treating obesity. If obesity could be treated, then Type 2 diabetics—and many Type 1 diabetics who develop insulin resistance after age forty—could experience fewer complications from diabetes, such as cardiovascular disease, degenerative arthritis caused by being overweight, and pulmonary complications, such as sleep apnea. Treating the underlying cause of diabetes, in this case obesity, could prevent or delay a diagnosis of the disease in a lot of patients.

New Ways to Deliver Insulin

Finding ways to coax the body into producing its own insulin is the miracle that scientists and people who have diabetes long to see. But other research efforts are underway that will make diabetes a more easily managed disease. One area of research is the quest to develop new methods administering insulin. Daily injections with needles and syringes work well, but for some patients are painful. And the pump works well if you are capable of setting your insulin dosages and can afford the cost of buying one. These new insulin delivery devices offer the promise of less invasive, less costly techniques.

Insulin Inhalers

Like an asthma inhaler, an insulin inhaler would administer insulin via the mouth and into the lungs. The fast-acting insulin would come in the form of a liquid or powder and would be taken at meal time. But the amount of insulin your body actually absorbs might vary, depending on your age and respiratory condition. Possible side effects include a mild cough, decreased pulmonary function, and scarring of the lungs. There are also questions about the long-term use and safety of insulin inhalers.

Mouth Sprays

An aerosol spray releases insulin into the oral cavity, allowing you to absorb insulin through your cheeks and the back of your mouth instead of the lungs. At the moment, there are both a fast-acting and long-acting mouth spray insulin under development.

Insulin Pills

Popping a pill would seem an easy way to take insulin, but its breakdown in the digestive system has made oral delivery of insulin a challenge. Because insulin pills do not make it into the liver and the bloodstream, they are unable to do their job of allowing glucose to enter body cells for conversion into energy. Researchers are looking for ways to prevent the oral insulin from breaking down in the digestive tract.

Insulin Patch

Scientists are looking at the prospect of applying a simple patch onto the skin as a way to get your insulin. The patch would administer basal insulin—the kind you need throughout the day to stabilize blood glucose—through microscopic holes that you first make on your skin. Once applied, a patch could be left on for twelve to twenty-four hours.

New Glucose Monitoring Devices

Diabetics who don't like the fingerstick method of monitoring their blood glucose might be glad to hear that new, less invasive devices for monitoring blood glucose are in development.

In the future, diabetics may be able to detect blood glucose via a patch that can draw glucose from the fluids in your skin. Or maybe they'll be able to use near infrared light beams to detect the presence of blood sugar in skin tissue. The new technologies would eliminate the use of the fingerstick, which some patients find painful.

Clinical Trials: Are They a Good Idea?

Before any treatment can be approved by the FDA for mass distribution, several research studies are required to prove that the treatment is safe and effective. That's where clinical trials come in. Clinical trials, also called clinical studies, are carefully conducted research studies done in human volunteers to answer specific questions about a treatment or therapy. The treatment might be a new vaccine, drug, medical device, or procedure. The trials are done in three separate phases after research in laboratories produces promising results in animals. The goal is then to find out how the new therapy or procedure will work in people, how much they need to take for it to have a positive effect, and whether the treatment is both safe and effective. In addition to drug treatments, clinical trials look at methods of prevention, diagnosis, screening, and ways to improve the quality of life.

Several different kinds of organizations are involved in doing clinical trials, including doctors, medical institutions, pharmaceutical companies, foundations, government agencies, and others. The trials are done in various settings, ranging from a small doctor's office to a large university or hospital. All clinical trials are governed by an Institutional Review Board made up of an independent committee of physicians, community advocates, and others who oversee the ethics of the research, ensuring that the rights of the participants are protected and reviewing the research on a periodic basis.

As a diabetic, you might consider participating in a clinical trial of a diabetes treatment or procedure. By doing so, you might gain access to a medication that is not widely available. You may also enjoy medical care at leading health-care facilities. Some people may feel they've exhausted all other options. For others, the altruism of contributing to science and the development of treatments for the disease may be enough to convince them to join.

Before you can participate however, you have to make sure you qualify for the trial. Researchers must set eligibility requirements, or trial guidelines. Some people may be excluded because of age, gender, the stage of the disease, and other medical conditions. Some trials want candidates who have a certain condition. Others require healthy people. After meeting with the doctors and nurses involved in the trial, you will need to sign an informed consent document that says you understand the risks and benefits of participating. Volunteering to participate does not guarantee that you will be included.

Being part of a clinical trial does involve risks. Some participants might be given a placebo, or inactive treatment, which is used to gauge the treatment's effectiveness. If you do receive the treatment, you may experience unpleasant, even life-threatening side effects. You might also have to endure frequent visits to the testing site, treatments, and hospital stays. And for all the time and energy you invest, you may also find that the treatment has no beneficial effect on your condition.

To Help You Decide
According to www.clinicaltrials.gov, a website of the National Institutes of Health, there are several things you should know before you decide to participate in a clinical trial:

- What is the purpose of the study?
- Who is going to be in the study?
- Why do researchers believe the new treatment being tested may be effective?
- Has it been tested before?
- What kinds of tests and treatments are involved?
- How do the possible risks, side effects, and benefits in the study compare with what I'm currently taking?
- How might this trial affect my life?
- How long will the trial last?
- Will hospitalization be required?
- Who will pay for the treatment?
- Will I be reimbursed for other expenses?
- What type of long-term follow-up care is part of the study?
- How will I know if the treatment is working?
- Will I see the results of the trial?
- Who will be in charge of my care?

Before you make any final decision, talk to your physician, family members, and friends. Balance the positives with the negatives and gather information about specific trials. If you think you'd like to participate, check out www.clinicaltrials.gov, a website that has information about more than 8,000 clinical trials being done primarily in the U.S. and Canada, but also in some foreign sites. You might also contact doctors, hospitals, or health-care organizations for information.

A Final Note

Modern medicine has made great strides in the field of diabetes research. Less than a century ago, a diagnosis of diabetes was a death sentence. Today, with so much research underway, diabetics live with the hope for a cure and the dream of being freed from the cumbersome chores of monitoring blood glucose, injecting insulin, and taking oral medications.

But until that cure is discovered, your health remains in your hands. Diabetes is a chronic disease that requires constant vigilance, which means among other things, keeping your blood glucose in a normal range, trying to maintain a healthy weight, eating well, and exercising. Taking good care of your health will help you avoid and minimize the complications of this disease and ensure a higher quality of life. How you choose to live with diabetes will shape your future as well as the future of those around you. We hope you choose to live wisely.

CHAPTER FIFTEEN

Diabetes Resources

If you were recently diagnosed with diabetes or are trying to figure out how to manage some aspect of your care, you'll be happy to know that there's a wealth of information available on the topic of diabetes. Diabetes comes up frequently in consumer media such as television, newspapers, and magazines, and is also a popular research subject in medical journals. In this chapter, we provide you with a list of good resources for reliable information.

American Diabetes Association
1701 North Beauregard Street
Alexandria, VA 22311
1-800-DIABETES (1-800-342-2383)
On-line: www.diabetes.org

American Association of Diabetes Educators
100 W. Monroe, Suite 400
Chicago, IL 60603
1-800-338-3633
On-line: www.aadenet.org; or email aade@aadenet.org

American Dietetic Association
120 South Riverside Plaza, Suite 2000
Chicago, IL 60606-6995
1-800-877-1600
On-line: www.eatright.org

American Heart Association
National Center
7272 Greenville Avenue
Dallas, TX 75231
1-800-242-8721
On-line: www.americanheart.org

American Stroke Association
National Center
7272 Greenville Avenue
Dallas TX 75231
1-888-478-7653
On-line: www.strokeassociation.org

Hypoglycemia Support Foundation, Inc.
PO BOX 451778
Sunrise, FL 33345
On-line: www.hypoglycemia.org
email: rruggiero@hypoglycemia.org

Joslin Diabetes Center
One Joslin Place
Boston, MA 02215
(617) 732-2400
On-line: www.joslin.harvard.edu

Juvenile Diabetes Research Foundation International
120 Wall Street
New York, NY 10005-4001
1-800-533-CURE (2873)
Fax: (212) 785-9595
On-line: www.jdrf.org or by email: info@jdrf.org

National Institute of Diabetes and Digestive and Kidney Diseases
National Diabetes Information Clearinghouse
1 Information Way
Bethesda, MD 20892-3560
1-800-860-8747
On-line: www.niddk.nih.gov

National Diabetes Education Program, a program of the NIDDK
One Diabetes Way
Bethesda, MD 20814-9692
1-800-438-5383
On-line: www.ndep.nih.gov; or write to: ndep@info.nih.gov

Helpful Websites
The Internet is a wonderful source of information about diabetes—if you know where to look. In addition to the websites provided by the organizations and agencies above, here are some others recommended by the ADA:

Centers for Disease Control and Prevention:
www.cdc.gov/health/diabetes.htm

Children with Diabetes, an on-line community:
www.childrenwithdiabetes.org

Diabetes Monitor:
www.diabetesmonitor.com

International Diabetes Federation:
www.idf.org/home

MEDline plus Health Information
from the National Library of Medicine:
www.nlm.nih.gov/medlineplus/

WebMD:
www.diabetes.com

GLOSSARY

Below is a list of words commonly associated with diabetes. Please note that the glossary includes medication categories for diabetes, but not for other disorders.

Alpha-glucosidase inhibitors: Drugs that work by slowing the digestion and absorption of carbohydrates through the small intestine, causing a less exaggerated spike in blood glucose after meals. The drugs also help lower the levels of glycated hemoglobin. The two drugs in this category are miglitol (Glyset) and acarbose (Precose).

Arrhythmias: Abnormal heart rhythms that can bring on palpitations, lightheadedness, or fainting.

Atherosclerosis: The buildup of fatty substances on the walls of the arteries, causing blood vessels to narrow.

Autoimmunity: A condition in which the immune system attacks its own healthy cells.

Automatic injector: A device that automatically shoots insulin into your skin using a needle.

Autonomic neuropathy: Nerve damage in the autonomic nervous system that affects bodily functions such as digestion, heart rate, breathing, and bladder control.

Basal: The steady amount of insulin administered throughout the day that helps keep blood glucose levels stable between meals.

Beta cells: The production centers for insulin located in the Islets of Langerhans in the pancreas.

Biguanides: A class of drugs that works by limiting the amount of stored glucose released by the liver and decreasing the amount of sugar that gets absorbed into your intestines. Metformin (Glucophage) is a biguanide.

Blood glucose monitor or meter: A computerized device that measures blood glucose levels from a test strip.

Body mass index (BMI): A measurement of how much of your body weight is fat. The BMI is used to help determine your risk for health problems associated with weight.

Bolus: A dosage of insulin given before or after meals to handle increases in blood glucose levels that occurs with the intake of food.

Brittle diabetes: Frequent highs and lows in blood glucose levels.

Carbohydrates: A macronutrient that provides the primary source of energy and comes in the form of simple and complex.

Carbohydrate counting: A dietary strategy for diabetics that tallies the amount of carbohydrates eaten in a meal or snack.

Cardiovascular disease: A broad category of diseases that are linked to how efficiently your heart pumps blood (cardio) or how well your blood circulates through your blood vessels (vascular).

Cataracts: An eye condition that commonly occurs with advancing age in which the lenses of your eyes become cloudy.

Certified diabetes educator: Health-care professionals specially trained to teach about diabetes. A CDE must pass a national test, with re-certification exams required every five years.

Charcot's joints: A rare but debilitating foot deformity caused by nerve damage to the feet. The condition occurs when joints are repeatedly fractured and eventually damaged.

Cholesterol: A naturally occurring waxy fat-like substance involved in making and repairing cell membranes, and producing hormones such as estrogen and testosterone. Cholesterol also comes from foods such as meat, butter, and cheese.

Clinical trial: A research study done with human volunteers to determine the safety, efficacy, and risks involved with a specific therapy.

Coronary artery disease (CAD): A buildup of fatty deposits that occurs in an artery leading to the heart, potentially damaging the heart muscle.

Data management system: A computerized device that measures your blood glucose and stores information about date, time, reading, insulin, exercise, and diet. Some systems will allow you to download the information onto your computer or your doctor's computer.

Dawn phenomenon: High blood glucose that occurs in the morning when growth hormones suppress the effects of insulin.

DCCT: The Diabetes Control and Complications Trial, which was completed in 1983. The study involved 1,441 people and showed that intensive control of blood glucose levels could lower the risks for complications.

Depression: A serious disorder that affects mood and causes a chronic state of sadness, despair, and helplessness.

D-phenylalanine: A new category of drugs that works by stimulating the rapid production of insulin needed right after a meal. Nateglinide (Starlix) is the only drug in this category that's been approved for use.

Dermatologist: A medical doctor trained in treating skin problems.

Diabetic ketoacidosis (DKA): A rare but potentially fatal condition caused by inadequate amounts of insulin. Without enough insulin, the liver gets the signal to break down fat for energy, which produces ketones. Untreated, DKA can lead to seizures, coma, and death.

Diabetes: A metabolic disorder that causes a malfunction of the body's ability to use the energy in food.

Diabetologists: Medical doctors who have a special interest in treating diabetes.

Dialysis: A treatment for end-stage renal disease in which the blood is cleansed of impurities, without removing the blood cells you need.

Diplopia: Double vision in diabetes that occurs when the blood vessels and nerves controlling the movement of the eyes are damaged.

Edmonton Protocol: A Canadian study that used a special regimen of immunosuppressive drugs for islet cell transplants.

Endocrinologists: Medical doctors who specialize in diseases affecting the endocrine system, such as diabetes.

End-stage renal disease: Severe kidney damage that impairs the functioning of the kidneys.

Entrapment neuropathies: A type of mononeuropathy that produces compression, pressure, or damage and can result in mechanical damage to a body part. One example is carpal tunnel syndrome.

Erectile dysfunction: The inability to have or maintain an erection, making intercourse impossible. Also called impotence.

Exchange system: A method of planning meals for diabetics that uses lists of six food groups that are similar in calories, carbohydrates, protein, and fat content.

Exenatide LAR: A long-acting release formula of the drug Exenatide. See Synthetic exendin-4 (Exenatide).

Exercise physiologist: Scientifically trained professionals who can help clients devise a safe, effective exercise program.

Fasting plasma glucose test: A blood test done after an overnight fast that determines whether a patient has high blood sugar.

Fats: Macronutrients that play a critical role in the brain and nervous system. Fats come in two basic forms, saturated and unsaturated.

Follicular phase: A phase of a woman's monthly cycle that begins with menstruation and ends with ovulation.

Gestational diabetes: A condition of diabetes that occurs during pregnancy.

Glaucoma: A condition in which the fluid in the eye builds up and causes excessive pressure that can lead to retinal damage. Glaucoma is more common among diabetics than healthy people.

Glucagon: A fast-acting hormone made in the pancreas that halts the liver's release of insulin and promotes the release of glucose. Glucagon is available by prescription as a treatment for hypoglycemia.

Glucagon-like peptide 1 (GLP-1): A new medication that is being investigated as a treatment for both Type 1 and Type 2 diabetes.

Glucose: A sugar derived primarily from the carbohydrates you eat. Once digested, it travels into the bloodstream, where the hormone insulin lets it into body cells for conversion into energy. In people who have diabetes, the cells don't respond to the insulin or the body doesn't produce enough of it.

GlucoWatch Biographer: A monitoring device worn like a wrist watch that uses a sensor to detect blood glucose levels in perspiration.

Glycated hemoglobin levels: The amount of hemoglobin molecules in red blood cells that are glycated, or coated in sugar, measured by the HbA1C test. The more glucose you have in your blood, the more glycated hemoglobin you will have. Healthy people usually have a 5 percent reading. Diabetics should strive for a reading of 6.5 percent or less. The amount of glycated hemoglobin in your blood gives you a bigger picture of how well you are controlling your blood glucose levels.

Glycemic index: A measuring system that gauges the rate in which sugar is released into your bloodstream. The higher the index rating, the faster the food sends sugar into your blood.

Heart attack: A potentially fatal reaction that occurs when the blood supply to the heart muscle is severely reduced or stopped. The cutoff of blood flow is the result of a blockage in one of the coronary arteries that supplies blood to the heart (also known as a myocardial infarction).

Hemodialysis: A type of dialysis that involves being hooked up to a machine at a clinic, which acts like an artificial kidney. The blood is removed from an artery, circulated through the machine, then returned to the body through a vein.

High-density lipoproteins (HDLs): A lipoprotein often called "the good cholesterol," that scoops up excess cholesterol and brings it to the liver, where it is broken down and eliminated.

HLA genes: Genes responsible for the functioning of human leukocyte antigens that have been linked to Type 1 diabetes, namely HLA-DR3 and HLA-DR4.

Hyperglycemia: A condition in which blood glucose levels rise too high, causing fatigue, excessive thirst, frequent urination, and dehydration. Blood sugar is generally 250 mg/dl or higher in hyperglycemia.

Hyperglycemic hyperosmolar non-ketotic coma (HHNC): A condition in which blood sugar levels get dangerously high. Also called hyperglycemic hyperosomolar state (HHS).

Hypoglycemia: A condition in which blood glucose levels fall too low, causing nervousness, irritability, shakiness, and extreme hunger. The condition is common among patients who use intensive therapy to manage their diabetes. Hypoglycemia usually occurs when blood sugars fall below 50 to 60 mg/dl, but can vary from one person to the next.

Hypoglycemia unawareness: A condition in which a person is unable to detect the symptoms of hypoglycemia.

Hyperfiltration: An early condition in diabetes in which the kidneys are working harder than usual.

Hypertrophy: The overgrowth of fat cells that produces lumpy looking skin caused by the injection of insulin.

Impotence: The inability to have or maintain an erection, making intercourse impossible. Also called erectile dysfunction.

Infusers: A device that reduces the number of times you poke yourself with a needle. Infusers are tiny catheters inserted under the skin that stay in place with tape for up to three days. Whenever you need insulin, you inject the needle into the infuser. Although less painful, the infuser can raise the risk for local infection.

Injection sites: The location on the body where insulin is injected. Common injection sites include the abdomen, upper and outer thighs, backs of the upper arms, the thighs, or the buttocks.

Insulin: A hormone produced in the pancreas that is responsible for moving glucose from the blood into body cells for the conversion into energy. In healthy people, insulin is secreted after a meal. Insulin also plays a role in the storage of extra glucose by the liver. When insulin levels are high, the liver accepts and stores extra glucose in the form of glycogen. When insulin levels are low, the liver releases glycogen into the blood as sugar for extra energy. The constant ebb and flow of glycogen from the liver also helps keep blood sugar at normal levels.

Insulin analogs: Long-acting insulin that provide a more constant release of the hormone into the fatty tissue. Glargine (Lantus) U-100 insulin, the first insulin analog, behaves much like an insulin pump does and may be administered once a day.

Intensive insulin therapy: A method of managing diabetes with the goal of mimicking the way your body naturally secretes insulin. The therapy involves adjusting insulin to accommodate everyday changes in diet, activity level, and blood glucose levels. It is often recommended for Type 1 diabetics and women with gestational diabetes, who need to have tight control of blood sugars.

Intermediate-acting insulin: A type of insulin that has an onset time of one to three hours, peaks at eight hours, and can last as long as twenty hours. Examples include Humulin N and Novolin.

Islet cell transplants: The transplanting of insulin-producing cells into people who have Type 1 diabetes as a way to restore function to damaged beta cells.

Islet neogenesis associated protein: A gene under scientific study that may be able to aid in the regeneration of insulin-producing cells in the pancreas. Also called INGAP.

Islets of Langerhans: The production centers of insulin located in the pancreas.

Jaundice: A condition in newborns caused by excess amounts of bilirubin, a byproduct of the breakdown of red blood cells. The condition is more common in babies born to mothers with diabetes and causes a yellowish hue in the baby's skin.

Jet injectors: A needle-less device that injects insulin into the skin.

Ketones: A product produced by the body when it breaks down fats for energy. Poorly managed glucose levels may result in ketones in the urine and lead to diabetic ketoacidosis.

Kidney disease: A complication of diabetes caused by blockages in the tiny blood vessels of the kidneys, interfering with their ability to filter toxins and retain protein, and causing leakage.

Kidney failure: A condition in which the kidneys no longer filter toxins from the blood and cannot remove proteins from it.

Kidney transplant: A treatment for kidney failure in which a failed kidney is surgically removed and replaced with a healthy one from a living donor, or someone who has recently died.

Lancet: A small needle that draws blood with a quick prick of the finger.

Lipid profile: A test that tells you how much cholesterol is circulating in your blood. The profile should include readings of total cholesterol, low-density lipoprotein (LDLs), and high-density lipoproteins (HDLs), as well as triglycerides.

Lipoatrophy: Dents in the skin near the injection site, caused by the disappearance of fatty tissue under the skin.

Lipohypertrophy: A buildup of fat deposits caused by using the same injection site over and over again.

Long-acting insulin: A type of insulin that takes longer to go into effect. Some brands peak between eight and twelve hours, but others may have no peak time. The insulin may remain in effect for anywhere from twenty-four to thirty-six hours.

Low-density lipoproteins: Often called the "bad cholesterol," LDLs are responsible for spreading cholesterol throughout the body, where they can build up on blood vessel walls.

Luteal phase: A phase of a woman's monthly cycle that begins at ovulation and ends with menstruation.

Macrosomia: A condition that may be caused by a mother having diabetes in which a baby grows unusually large in utero.

Macular edema: Swelling of the macula of the eye caused by fluid leaking from the cells of the retina. The condition causes blurring, distortion, and difficulties seeing blue and yellow colors, and may lead to vision loss.

Meglitinides: A drug class that works by stimulating the beta cells to release more insulin, which helps reduce postprandial blood glucose elevation. The drugs react directly in response to a meal. Repaglinide (Prandin) is the only drug in this category approved for use in the U.S.

Menstruation: The monthly shedding of the uterine lining that occurs if an egg is unfertilized.

Mental-health professional: A health-care provider who specializes in treating emotional and mental problems. They may work as social workers, psychologists, psychiatrists, or counselors.

Microalbuminuria: An early sign of kidney disease marked by small amounts of protein in the urine.

MiniMed Continuous Glucose Monitoring System: A blood glucose monitoring device that uses a small catheter inserted just below the skin to collect liquid that is then passed through a biosensor.

Mononeuropathy: Damage to a single nerve or group of nerves, caused by a blockage in a blood vessel that supplies that nerve or nerves. Also called focal neuropathy.

National Institute of Diabetes and Digestive and Kidney Diseases: A branch of the National Institutes of Health that specializes in diabetes and other disorders of the endocrine system (NIDDK).

Nephrologist: A medical doctor who specializes in the treatment of the kidneys.

Neuropathy: A complication of diabetes that involves damage to the nerves.

Obesity: A condition characterized by excess amounts of body fat and technically defined as having a body mass index of thirty or higher.

Ophthalmologists: Medical doctors trained to detect and treat eye problems with surgery or medications.

Optometrists: Professionals specializing in vision health who can detect eye problems caused by diabetes, but cannot do surgery to correct them.

Oral glucose tolerance test: A tool for diagnosing diabetes that uses a drink laced with high amounts of glucose.

Ovulation: The release of an egg that occurs in a woman's menstrual cycle.

Pen injectors: Devices for injecting insulin that resemble pens.

Peripheral neuropathy: Damage to the peripheral nervous system, which includes the arms, hands, legs, and feet. Also called distal symmetric polyneuropathy.

Peritoneal dialysis: A type of dialysis in which a solution called dialysate is inserted into your abdominal cavity to collect waste. After a certain interval, the solution is drained, then repeated again every four to six hours.

PMS: A common term for premenstrual syndrome that occurs in women in the week before their period. Symptoms include irritability, fatigue, cramps, bloating, and cravings for unhelathy foods.

Podiatrist: A medical doctor who specializes in the treatment of feet and has a Doctor of Podiatric Medicine (DPM) degree.

PPAR gamma: A gene that's been identified as a marker for developing Type 2 diabetes that may also help prevent the disease in obese people.

Pramlintide acetate (Symlin): A synthetic version of the human hormone amylin and first in a class of medications known as amylinomimetic agents or amylin receptor agonists.

Pre-diabetes: A condition characterized by blood glucose levels above 100 mg/dl, but less than 126 mg/dl.

Preeclampsia: Excessively high blood pressure in pregnancy. Also called toxemia.

Protein: A macronutrient made up of amino acids that aids in the building and repair of body cells. Protein comes from several sources, including meat, eggs, dairy, legumes, nuts, and seeds.

Proteinuria: A condition characterized by large amounts of protein in the urine.

Pump: A small portable gadget used to infuse insulin into the body. Pumps imitate the action of insulin in healthy people by delivering a steady dose of insulin all through the day (basal) and a larger jolt of insulin whenever blood glucose levels rise (bolus). The pump uses a small needle inserted in the skin beneath fatty tissue and taped into place. The needle is attached to a catheter that connects to the pump, where the insulin is stored.

Random plasma glucose test: A test that uses samples of blood drawn shortly after eating or drinking to test for diabetes.

Rapid-acting insulin: Insulin that has an onset time of fifteen minutes, with peak action at thirty to ninety minutes. The effect typically lasts three to five hours. Examples include Humalog (lispro) and Novolog (aspart). The fast action means patients can easily time their insulin to their meals.

Registered dietitian (RD): Health-care professionals trained to understand the chemistry of food and nutrition who can help diabetics create a healthy meal plan. An RD at the end of the name means the person has met the standards set by the American Dietetic Association and passed a national credentialing exam.

Regular (short-acting) insulin: A type of insulin that goes into action in 30 to 60 minutes, peaks between 50 and 120 minutes, and can last from 5 to 8 hours. Examples include Humulin R and Novolin R.

Retinopathy: A medical condition that occurs when blood vessels that fortify the retina, the part of the eye that produces visual images, is damaged. Retinopathy is a complication of diabetes.

Self-monitoring of blood glucose (SMBG): A critical component in a patient's diabetes care in which a diabetic checks blood glucose levels. The information helps the patient understand what affects his blood glucose levels, and how it might be affected by insulin, medications, exercise, and diet, and also how well blood glucose is being controlled.

Serum creatinine: A chemical waste product that appears in high concentrations in the urine if kidney function is impaired.

Short-acting (regular) insulin: A type of insulin that goes into action in 30 to 60 minutes, peaks between 50 and 120 minutes, and can last from 5 to 8 hours. Examples include Humulin R and Novolin R.

Somogyi phenomenon: A rapid shift from low to high levels of blood glucose that occurs when the body responds to hypoglycemia with a surge in blood glucose levels. The condition may be triggered by eating too many carbohydrates in response to hypoglycemia.

Stem cells: Undifferentiated embryonic stem cells that may be grown into other body cells such as pancreatic beta cells. Research suggests stem cells may provide a cure for Type 1 diabetes.

Stroke: A physical reaction that occurs when the blood supply to the brain is cut off.

Sulfonylureas: Sulfur-containing medications used to treat diabetes that work by stimulating the beta cells in the pancreas to produce and release more insulin. Drugs in this category include Dymelor, Diabinese, Glucamide, Amaryl, Glucotrol, Diabeta, Glynase, Micronase, Tolinase, and Orinase.

Synthetic exendin-4 (Exenatide): The first of a new class of medications for Type 2 diabetes called incretin mimetic agents.

Syringe: A method of injecting insulin that consists of a needle, barrel, and plunger. It works by drawing insulin out of a bottle, and then injecting the insulin under fatty tissue in your skin.

Test strip: A chemically treated piece of paper used to test for glucose in a monitor.

Thiazolidinediones: Drugs that work by making body tissues more sensitive to insulin. In cases of prolonged hyperglycemia, they help promote the production of insulin. Also called glitazones, these drugs include rosiglitazone (Avandia) and pioglitazone (Actos). A third drug, troglitazone (Rezulin) was removed from the market in 2000 after several cases of liver failure were linked to its use.

Transient ischemic attacks (TIAs): Brief episodes in which the brain ceases functioning because of a temporary deprivation of oxygen due to blocked blood vessels. If TIAs last longer than an hour, the event is called a stroke.

Triglycerides: The primary form of fat in food and the body's stored form of fat. High levels are said to be linked to cardiovascular disease.

Type 1 diabetes: A condition in which the body attacks healthy insulin-producing cells in the pancreas. Without insulin, the glucose can't get inside the cells and instead is left to linger in the bloodstream. Having too much blood glucose is diabetes. Formerly called insulin-dependent diabetes or juvenile diabetes.

Type 2 diabetes: A condition in which body cells become resistant to the effects of insulin or in which the pancreas stops making enough insulin, causing excess glucose in the blood. Formerly called non-insulin-dependent diabetes.

Urinary tract infections: A bacterial infection of the urinary tract that can become more common in diabetics.

BIBLIOGRAPHY

American Diabetes Association Complete Guide to Diabetes, 3rd edition, American Diabetes Association, Alexandria, V.A., 2002.

Collazo-Clavell, Maria, M.D. (editor in chief). *Mayo Clinic on Managing Diabetes*, Mason Crest Publishers, Broomall, P.A., 2002.

Duyff, Roberta, M.S., R.D., CFCS. *The American Dietetic Association's Complete Food & Nutrition Guide*, Chronimed Publishing, Minneapolis, M.N., 1996.

Goldmann, David R., M.D. (editor), *American College of Physicians Complete Home Medical Guide*, DK Publishing, Inc., New York, N.Y., 1999.

Hammerly, Milton, M.D. and Cheryl Kimball. *What to Do When the Doctor Says It's PCOS*, Fair Winds Press, Gloucester, M.A., 2003.

Johnson, Robert V., M.D. (editor in chief). *Mayo Clinic Complete Book of Pregnancy & Baby's First Year*, William and Morrow and Co., New York, N.Y, 1994.

Milchovich, Sue K., R.N., B.S.N., C.D.E. and Barbara Dunn Long, R.D. *Diabetes Mellitus: A Practical Handbook*, 8th edition, Bull Publishing, Boulder, CO, 2003.

Physicians Committee for Responsible Medicine with Patricia Bertron, R.D. *Healthy Eating for Life to Prevent and Treat Diabetes*, John Wiley & Sons, Inc., New York, N.Y., 2002.

Powers, Maggie, M.S. R.D., C.D.E. *Eating Right When You Have Diabetes*, John Wiley & Sons, Inc., Hoboken, N.J, 2003.

Smolin, Lori and Mary B. Grosvenor, *Nutrition Science and Applications*, Saunders College Publishing, a division of Harcourt Brace College Publishers, Orlando, F.L., 1994.

Touchette, Nancy, PhD., *The Diabetes Problem Solver*, American Diabetes Association, Alexandria, V.A., 1999.

Warshaw, Hope, MMSc, R.D., C.D.E. and Karmeen Kulkarni, M.S., R.D., C.D.E. *Complete Guide to Carbohydrate Counting*, American Diabetes Association, Alexandria, V.A., 2001.

Articles

Adams, Amy. "Researchers look to stem cell techniques to better treat diabetes," *Stanford Report*, Jan. 8, 2003.

Alexander, CM et al. "NCEP-defined metabolic syndrome, diabetes, and prevalance of coronary heart disease among NHANES III participants age 50 years and older," *Diabetes*, May 2003, v52 n5 p1210.

American Diabetes Association, "Type 2 Diabetes in children and adolescents," *Diabetes Care*, March 2000, v23 n3 p381.

Amschler, Denise, "The alarming increase of type 2 diabetes in children," *Journal of School Health*, Jan. 2002 v72 n1, p39.

Beheme M.T. et al. "Glucagon-like peptide 1 improved glycemic control in type 1 diabetes," BMC Endocrine Disorders, April 10, 2003, http://www.biomedcentral.com/1472-6823/3/3.

Black SA et al. "Depression predicts increased incidence of adverse health outcomes in older Mexican Americans with type 2 diabetes," *Diabetes Care*, Oct. 2003, v26 n10 p2822.

Center for Genome Research. "Scientists identify a single nucleotide polymorphism (SNP) responsible for increased risk of diabetes," press release, Aug. 27, 2000.

Ehlers, MR et al. "Recombinant glucagon-like peptide-1 (7-36) amide) lowers fasting serum glucose in a broad spectrum of patients with type 2 diabetes," *Hormone and Metabolic Research*, Oct. 2003, v35 n10 p611.

"Exubera inhaled insulin for type 1 and 2 diabetes," www.drugdevelopment technology.com/project

Gardner, Amanda. "Liver Cells converted into pancreatic ones, scientific coaxing holds promise for diabetes," Healthscout.com, Jan. 31, 2003.

Holz, GG and Chepurny, OG. "Glucagon-like peptide-1 synthetic analogs:new therapeutic agents for use in the treatment of diabetes mellitus," *Current Medicinal Chemistry*, Nov. 2003, v10 n22 p2471.

Joslin Diabetes Center. "Patients with diabetes who have heart attacks fare better if they have had bypass surgery rather than angioplasty to treat heart disease," press release, April 2000, www.joslin.harvard.edu/news/bypassVangioplast.shtml.

Koh, EH et al. "Peroxisome proliferator-activated receptor (PPAR)-alpha activation prevents diabetes in OLETF rats: comparison with PPAR-gamma activation," *Diabetes*, Sept. 2003 v52 n9 p2331.

Rados, Carol. "Inside clinical trials, testing medical products in people," *FDA Consumer*, Sept.-Oct. 2003, www.fda.gov/fdac/features/2003/503_trial.html.

Shapiro, AMJ et al. "Islet transplantation in seven patients with type 1 diabetes mellitus using a glucocorticoid-free immunosuppressive regimen," *New England Journal of Medicine*, July 27, 2000, v343 n4 p230.

Slaughter, Adele, "Bret Michaels rocks the diabetes world," *USA Today*, July 1, 2002.

Mitchell, Jacqueline, "Stem Cells 101," May 28, 2002, www.pbs.org/saf/1209/features/stemcell2.htm, .

Watkins, Carol E. and Terri Kordella. "When Your Child is Diagnosed," *Diabetes Forecast*, Sept. 2003 v55 n9 p82.

Websites

www.aafp.org: American Academy of Family Physicians

www.acog.org: American College of Obstetricians and Gynecologists

www.americanheart.org: American Heart Association

www.amylin.com: Amylin Pharmaceuticals

www.childrenwithdiabetes.com: Children With Diabetes

www.clinicaltrials.gov: a service of the National Institutes of Health

www.diabetes.org: American Diabetes Association

www.diabeteseducator.org: American Association of Diabetes Educators

www.diabetesmonitor.com: Diabetes Monitor.com

www.diabetesnet.com: The Diabetes Mall

www.diabetic-talk.org: Diabetic Talk.Org

www.drugdigest.org: Drug Digest

www.evms.edu: Strelitz Diabetes Institute at Eastern Virginia Medical School

www.fda.gov: U.S. Food and Drug Administration

www.glucophagexr.com: Information about Glucophage XR by Bristol-Myers Squibb Co.

www.healthtouch.com: Healthtouch Online, the Diabetes Place

www.insulin-free.org: Insulin-Free World Foundation

www.um-jmh.org/HealthLibrary/meds/Sulfonylureas.html: Jackson Health System

www.jdrf.org: Juvenile Diabetes Research Foundation

www.joslin.harvard.edu: Joslin Center

www.mayoclinic.com: Mayo Clinic

www.news.wisc.edu/packages/stemcells/facts.html#4: Embryonic stem cells, research at University of Wisconsin-Madison.

www.niddk.nih.gov: National Institute of Diabetes and Digestive and Kidney Diseases (NIDDK)

www.nimh.nih.gov: National Institute of Mental Health

www.tcoyd.org: Taking Control of Your Diabetes

www.zetia.com: Information about Zetia from Merck/Schering Plough Pharmaceuticals

INDEX

in children, 226–28
genetics and, 21
increasing incidence of, 11–12, 226–28
prevention of, 227–28
risk factors for, 21–23
tyramine, 211
TZDs. *See* thiazolidinediones

U
unsaturated fats, 68
urinary tract infections, 158, 164, 177, 190, 264
urination, frequent, 17, 24
urine tests, 26, 42–43

V
vacuum devices, 192
vaginal dryness, 189
vaginal infections, 164, 189–90
vasectomies, 196
vasodilators, 146
Viagra, 191–92
virus theory, 20
vision, blurred, 25
vitrectomy, 154

W
walking, 84
weakness, 25
websites, 249–50
weight, 40
weight gain, 25
weight loss
  cardiovascular disease and, 146
  counting calories and, 77–78
  helping children with, 228
  tips for, 79
  unexplained, 24

Y
yeast infections, 25, 164, 189–90

ACKNOWLEDGMENTS

First of all, I'd like to thank my editor Donna Raskin, whose faith in my abilities landed me the job of writing this book and allowed me to delve into what has become one of the most significant health problems of our time. I'd also like to thank Dr. Melvin Stjernholm for his careful perusal of my copy, always making sure to add the most up-to-date and pertinent information wherever needed—and even catching the occasional typo. His patients are fortunate to have him. In addition, I want to say thank you to all the people who were willing to share their stories about having diabetes. A special thank you goes out to my dear friend Jenny, who goes about the enormous task of raising two diabetic children without complaint and still has the joie de vivre she has had since seventh grade. She is an exemplary parent. Finally, I must thank Jeff, Samantha and Stephanie, my husband and daughters, who gave me their love and support as I toiled away. I am truly blessed to have them.

—Winnie Yu

ABOUT THE AUTHORS

WINNIE YU is a freelance writer focusing on health and parenting for national publications including *Woman's Day*, *Weight Watchers*, and *Parents*, in addition to the Web site www.drugdigest.org. Her work has also appeared in *Reader's Digest* and *The Wall Street Journal*, and she has contributed to several health book.

DR. STJERNHOLM is an endocrinologist who has been in private practice in Boulder, Colorado for the past thiry years. He is board certified in endocrinology, diabetes, and metabolism. He received his Doctor of Medicine cum laude from the University of Colorado School of Medicine, has been a teacher and educator to his peers, and holds an appointment as Clinical Professor of Medicine at the University of Colorado Health Sciences Center. Dr.Stjernholm started performing diabetes research as a medical student and since then has performed clinical research in the area of diabetes, lipids and hypertension. He believes the best way to prevent diabetes is to start treating obesity before it becomes the metabolic syndrome and diabetes.

Dr. Stjernholm is a member of the American Diabetes Association, past president of the Colorado Affiliate of the ADA, and is also a member of the Endocrine Society and the American Association of Clinical Endocrinologists. He received the outstanding physician award in the area of diabetes by the Colorado Diabetes Institute.

ALEXIS MUNIER is a writer and opera singer who was diagnosed with diabetes at age 13. She has traveled the world, performing in Colorado, Massachusetts, and California. She currently lives in Zurich.

Also available from Fair Winds Press

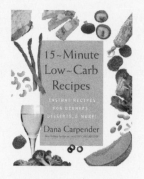

Yikes! It's 6:30 p.m., and you've just walked through the door after a long day at work, plus a couple of errands. You're tired, you're hungry—and before you can get your coat off, the family has started asking, "What's for dinner?"

In the past, you would have started boiling water for some quick mac-and-cheese, or warmed up a frozen pizza. Hungry and busy though you may be, you really don't want to trade your weight loss, high energy, and improved health for a quick-and-carb-y supper. What, of what, to do?

Sit down, relax, take a deep breath, and flip through *15-Minute Low-Carb Recipes*. You'll find dozens of wonderful family dishes that take no more than fifteen minutes to make, prep time included, with carbohydrate, fiber, and usable carb counts already calculated for you. What could be easier?

Dana Carpender appears frequently on national television and radio, and is the best-selling author of *500 Low-Carb Recipes, 15-Minute Low-Carb Recipes, The Low-Carb Barbecue Book, Dana Carpender's Carb Gram Counter,* and *How I Gave Up My Low-Fat Diet and Lost Forty Pounds.*

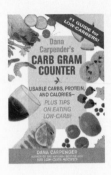

DANA CARPENDER'S
CARB GRAM COUNTER
by Dana Carpender
ISBN: 1-59233-077-0
$4.99 (£2.99)
Paperback; 320 pages
Available wherever books are sold

In this book you'll find a comprehensive directory of the total carbs, usable carbs, fiber, protein, and calorie amounts for countless different types of food. To make it easy to use, we've highlighted the usable carbs, so you can find the vital information at a glance. And to help you put more variety in your diet, we've also highlighted the foods with less than five grams of usable carbs per serving, so you can see what you may have been missing!

To help you maintain a low-carb diet happily and successfully for life, we've included the best low-carb tips. We've even put together lists of great low-carb snacks, low-carb treats, fast food meals, and more.

So grab this little book, and carry it in your pocket, purse, or briefcase—it's the low-carb tool you've been looking for!

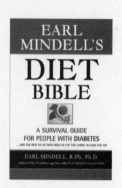

EARL MINDELL'S DIET BIBLE
by Earl Mindell, R.Ph., Ph.D.
ISBN: 1-931412-04-9
$14.95 (£9.99)
Paperback; 228 pages
Available wherever books are sold

Fine-tune your body for optimal weight, health, and energy!
You've trusted Dr. Mindell for more than twenty years for his revolutionary findings on natural supplements. So why trust anyone else when it comes to the groundbreaking Asian secret to regulating blood sugar safely and effectively? Insulin resistance and diabetes have reached epidemic levels in Western countries. In *Earl Mindell's Diet Bible*, you'll discover how they've developed and why prescription drugs aren't always the answer.

Some of the secrets Dr. Mindell Reveals:
• The simple evolutionary reason why fat won't make you fat—but bread will.
• Why the government doesn't want you to know the truth about carbo hydrate metabolism.
• Why the American Diabetes Association won't prevent ot cure Type 2 diabetes—and what will really save you from this epidemic!

In this book, Dr. Mindell tells the straight story about weight loss—what works, what doesn't, and how to melt those extra pounds for good.

Dr. Earl Mindell is the best-selling author of Earl Mindell's Vitamin Bible for the 21st Century and Earl Mindell's Herb Bible. A registered pharmacist and master herbalist, he holds a Ph.D. in nutrition and is a professor of nutrition at Pacific Western University in Los Angeles.